The XXL UK Low Carb Cookbook 2022-2023

Quick and Super-Delicious Low Carb Recipes to Kickstart Your New Healthy Lifestyle |14-Days Meal Plan Included

Karen C. Lee

Copyright© 2022 By Karen C. Lee All Rights Reserved

This book is copyright protected. It is only for personal use. You cannot amend, distribute, sell, use, quote or paraphrase any part of the content within this book, without the consent of the author or publisher.

Under no circumstances will any blame or legal responsibility be held against the publisher, or author, for any damages, reparation, or monetary loss due to the information contained within this book, either directly or indirectly.

Disclaimer Notice:

Please note the information contained within this document is for educational and entertainment purposes only. All effort has been executed to present accurate, up to date, reliable, complete information. No warranties of any kind are declared or implied. Readers acknowledge that the author is not engaged in the rendering of legal, financial, medical or professional advice. The content within this book has been derived from various sources. Please consult a licensed professional before attempting any techniques outlined in this book.

By reading this document, the reader agrees that under no circumstances is the author responsible for any losses, direct or indirect, that are incurred as a result of the use of the information contained within this document, including, but not limited to, errors, omissions, or inaccuracies.

Table of Contents

INTRODUCTION 1
    What Is Actually Low Carb? 2
        Low carb eating 2
        Low carb food list to avoid 4
        Other basic tips 4
    Health Benefits of a Low Carb Diet 4
        Lose weight 4
        Reverse type 2 diabetes 5
        A grateful gut 5
        Reduce sugar cravings 5
        Lowers the risk of heart disease 5
        Reduces risk of blood pressure 6
        Enhances brain health 6
        Reduces appetite 6
    What to Eat On a Low Carb Diet 6
        How to build your low-carb real food plate 6
        Low carb meal prep tips 7
        Low carb tips and guides 10
        14-day meal plan 11
CHAPTER 1 BREAKFASTS 14
    1. Sloppy Joe Sweet Potato Breakfast 14
    2. Air Fryer Avocado Baked Egg 14
    3. Keto Overnight Oats 15
    4. Keto Ham and Cheese Breakfast Biscuits 16
    5. Egg Mushroom Cups 16
    6. Fluffy Omelet with Cheese and Courgette 17
    7. Egg-Stuffed Avocado 18
    8. Meat Lovers Breakfast Pizza 18
    9. Breakfast Burrito Wrap with Bacon and Avocado 19
    10. Bacon and Spinach Egg Muffins 20
    11. Egg Casserole Hollandaise Sauce 21
    12. Keto Breakfast Bowl 22
    13. Keto Blueberry Pancakes 23
    14. Chia seed porridge 24
    15. Bacon Cauliflower Breakfast Skillet 24
    16. Keto Bacon and Egg Breakfast Bowls 25
    17. Low-Carb Sweet Potato Breakfast with Poached Egg 26
    18. Mango Kiwi Chia Seed Smoothie Bowl 26
CHAPTER 2 LUNCH 27
    1. Bacon Ranch ChickenSalad Cucumber Boats 27
    2. Greek Salmon Salad 28
    3. Chicken Taco Soup Recipe 29

4. Tuna Poke Salad 30
5. Rocket Salad with Crispy Prosciutto 31
6. Easy Braised Chicken Drumsticks in Tomatillo Sauce 32
7. Tomato Bisque with Basil Recipe 32
8. Chicken Broccoli Salad 33
9. Quick Buffalo Chicken Salad 33
10. Black Bean Avocado Salad 34
11. Citrus Prawns and Avocado Salad 34
12. Avocado Tuna Melt 35
13. Green Bean Salad 36
14. Chicken Club Sandwich 36
15. Stuffed Sweet Potatoes 37
16. Low-Carb & Keto Greek Chicken Bowls 38
17. Thai Chicken Lettuce Wraps 39
18. Spicy Thai Prawns Lettuce Wraps 40
19. Carne Asada Salad 41
20. Pan-Seared Filet Mignon Recipe with Herb Butter 42
21. Cheesy Taco Minced Beef & Cauliflower Rice Skillet 43
22. Easy Keto Pizza Chaffles 44
23. One Pot Low Carb and Keto Zuppa Toscana 44
24. Thai Peanut Salad 45
25. Minced Beef & Broccoli Casserole 46
26. Low Carb Steak Taco Bowl 47
27. Pineapple Teriyaki Meatballs 47
28. Vegetable Hash with Spicy Salmon Bites 48
29. Coriander Lime Grilled Prawns 49
30. Lemon Prawns with Garlic Olive Oil 50

CHAPTER 3 DINNER 51
1. Fluffy Omelet with Cheese and Courgette 51
2. Artichoke Chicken 51
3. Low Carb Hamburger Stroganoff 52
4. Quick Italian Eggs 53
5. Steak Kebabs with Chimichurri 53
6. Garlic Butter Pork Chops with Courgette 54
7. Pesto Salmon 55
8. Chipotle Air Fryer Chicken Thighs 56
9. Low Carb Aubergine Pizza 57
10. Mexican Taco Stuffed Courgette Boats 57
11. Crustless Cheesy Chicken and Asparagus Pie 58
12. Salmon in Roasted Pepper Sauce 59
13. Chicken Fried Cauliflower Rice 60
14. Orange Chicken Salad 61
15. Cuban Mojo Chicken 61
16. Coriander Lime Chicken 63

17. Baked Coconut Lime Chicken ... 64
18. Keto Cheesy Burger Stuffed Portobellos ... 65
19. Keto Chili ... 65
20. Low Carb Mushroom & Spinach Cauliflower Rice ... 66
21. Garlic Parmesan Brussels Sprouts with Bacon ... 67
22. Crustless Taco Pie ... 67
23. Chipotle Honey Chicken Skewers ... 68
24. Chicken Mushroom Soup ... 69
25. Spinach and Ricotta Hasselback Chicken ... 70
26. Caprese Chicken ... 70
27 Fried Steak and Asparagus Bundles ... 71
28. Spinach Stuffed Chicken Breasts ... 72
29. Pizza Flavored Keto Stuffed Tomato ... 73
30. Low Carb Goulash ... 74
31. Egg Roll In A Bowl ... 74
32. Red Pepper Egg-In-A-Hole ... 75

CHAPTER 4 SNACKS ... 76
1. Keto Skillet Cookie ... 76
2. Keto Strawberry Upside-Down Cake ... 76
3. Keto Cucumber Avocado and Pomegranate Salad ... 77
4. Low Carb Blueberry Cobbler ... 78
5. 3-ingredient No Bake Keto Peanut Butter Balls ... 78
6. Keto Jalapeno Poppers ... 79
7. Easy Strawberry Banana Smoothie Bowl ... 79
8. Keto Cauliflower Wings ... 80
9. Keto No Bake Peanut Butter And Jelly Bars ... 81

CHAPTER 5 APPETIZERS ... 82
1. Easy & Creamy Hot Crab Dip ... 82
2. Low Carb Nachos ... 82
3. Keto Buffalo Chicken Dip ... 83
4. Keto Jalapeño Poppers ... 83
5. Low Carb Deviled Eggs ... 84
6. Low Carb Rangoon ... 84
7. Low-carb Cheese Sticks ... 85
8. Easy Cheesy Courgette Breadsticks ... 85

Appendix 1 Measurement Conversion Chart ... 87
Appendix 2 Measurement Conversion Chart ... 88

INTRODUCTION

Low carb is becoming more and more popular. But what does it actually mean and how do you do it right? In this book we want to answer exactly these questions and give you a jump start by means of various recipes and a diet plan.

Low-carb diets limit carbohydrates, mostly pasta, bread, and sugary foods. Generally, we emphasize eating veggies and nutritious foods high in protein instead of carbohydrates. One of the three primary food groups that the body requires to function effectively is carbohydrates, often referred to as "carbs." Fats and protein usually make up the other two.

The body typically gets its energy from the carbs, which are converted by the body for immediate or future usage. However, when the body does not immediately require the consumed carbohydrates for energy, it just stores them in the liver and muscles for later use.

But if the body doesn't use the stored carbs, it turns them into fat. Many studies have shown low-carb diets promote weight loss and better health. Additionally, these diets have been widely used for years and are advocated by many healthcare experts.

The best part is that you typically don't need to use specific products or manage calories. All you have to do to have a balanced, nourishing, and satisfying diet is to consume whole foods.

Once carbs are reduced in the meals we consume, appetite is significantly reduced, thus, resulting in an automatic weight loss. My low-carb diet plan allows me to eat to fullness, feel satisfied, and still cut some weight.

There are no standardized amounts of carbohydrates that a low-carb meal must contain. Still, the number of carbs that individuals consume every day varies depending on their body type, age, activity levels, and sex.

I love cooking healthy foods and find delicious meals for lunch, breakfast, and dinner every day. So, I realized this has taken me back to natural and wholesome foods. In addition, there is concrete proof that the type of carbohydrates consumed (quality)—rather than quantity—affects an individual's health.

Diets high in fiber or slow to digest their carbs are healthier than foods heavy in sugars and refined grains. Individuals choosing a diet to address a specific health problem should have the diet customized to meet their particular requirements. For example, a diet containing roughly 40–50 percent carbs is advised for those with metabolic disorders.

Here, we will define a low-carb diet, talk about the benefits of eating low-carb if you have diabetes, and offer low-carb meal ideas to get you started if this is your typical diet.

Read this complete guide to learn how this eating style might help blood sugar control, weight loss, or other alleged health benefits.

What Is Actually Low Carb?

Low carb eating

Low carb eating entails reducing the number of carbohydrates consumed daily to less than 130 grams. As a result, the plate proportion of protein and fat is increased. Simply, we minimize the intake of starch and sugar, ensure we get enough or higher amounts of proteins, and enjoy meals with adequate natural fat.

Particular carbohydrate foods have essential fiber, minerals, and vitamins, thus, forming an integral part of a healthy diet. Although the fundamental purpose of a low-carb diet is weight loss, some diet forms go beyond that and pose some desirable health benefits, including reduction of risk of metabolic syndrome and type 2 diabetes.

There are many low carbohydrate foods, with each meal possessing distinct amounts and types of carbohydrates. Focus on eating foods like fish, eggs, and vegetables with natural fats but avoid starchy and sugary foods like rice, potatoes, bread, etc.

It would be best if you only ate when you're hungry and stopped once satisfied. So, it's just that simple; there is no essence in weighing the meal portions if counting calories.

Low-carb eating is different from no-carb eating! And, it's not an eating style for everyone. Thus, if you want this fantastic low-carb diet, ensure that you pick a meal plan that matches your food preferences, health goals, and personal lifestyle.

Why you might follow a low-carb diet

Following a diet with a reduced carb intake is determined by your specific goals and preferences. The primary reason people should follow a low-carb diet is that the body will burn the stored fat when it doesn't receive extra carbs, which promotes weight loss.

But, some people believe that restricting carbs in their diet results in less or no excess fat storage in the body. Low-carb diets have now gained mainstream acceptance, unlike some decades ago when they were highly controversial.

They are among the diets that help individuals drastically cut weight in the short term. Also, they are associated with improving health markers like blood pressure, blood sugar, and good cholesterol (HDL).

Other reasons to adopt the low-carb dieting style include:

- The need to change your overall eating habit
- The diet features enjoyable types and amounts of foods

However, we recommend checking with your healthcare provider before starting any weight loss dieting style. This is critical to people with underlying health conditions such as heart diseases and diabetes.

Typical food list for a low-carb diet

Your low-carb diet must be based on the natural, unprocessed foods below:

- Oils and fats—fish oil, olive oil, lard, butter, and coconut oil
- Meat—chicken, beef, pork, lamb, etc.
- Fruits—oranges, strawberries, apples, blueberries, and pears
- Fish—salmon, haddock, trout, etc.
- High-fat dairy—yogurt, cheese, butter, and doule cream
- Vegetables—broccoli, cauliflower, spinach, carrots, and others
- Seeds and nuts—almonds, sunflower seeds, and walnuts
- Eggs—pastured and omega-3 enriched eggs
- Beverages/drinks—water, tea, coffee, and sugar-free carbonated drinks such as sparkling water

You can include a few more carbs in your diet if you are super active, healthy, and don't need to cut extra weight. These include:

- Unrefined grains—quinoa, brown rice, and oats
- Tubers—sweet potatoes, potatoes, etc.
- Legumes—black beans, lentils, pinto beans, and many others
- Dry wines and organic dark chocolates may be taken in moderation

Low carb food list to avoid

These food groups need to be avoided at all times:

- Sugary foods—products that contain added sugar—soft drinks, candy, fruit juices, ice cream, and agave
- Starchy vegetables—limit all starchy vegetables if you're on a low-carb diet
- Trans-fats—partially or fully hydrogenated oils
- Refined grains—rice, wheat, barley, pasta, bread, and other processed cereals
- Low-fat foods—dairy products, crackers, etc. are low-fat foods but contain added sugar
- Highly processed foods—do not eat foods made in factories

Other basic tips

Despite the associated health benefits of a low-carb diet, you must be very careful. A drastic or sudden reduction in carbohydrates may cause temporary problems such as muscle cramps, constipation, and headache.

Severe carb restrictions will cause your body to burn down fats for energy, typically called ketosis. This is known to lead to weakness and fatigue. Other long-term side effects of restricting carbs in your diets include gastrointestinal disturbances and mineral/vitamin deficiencies.

In addition, pay attention to the fats and proteins you include in your diet. Unsaturated fats are recommended, but trans fats and saturated fats from animal sources should be limited since they increase the risk of heart diseases and certain cancers.

Health Benefits of a Low Carb Diet

Why should you think about consuming fewer carbs? There are numerous potential benefits for people of all ages, while there is rarely a reason for healthy children to follow a strict low-carb diet. Weight loss is the primary factor behind the low-carb diet and lifestyle popularity.

A low-carb strategy is not limited to that, though. In fact, the benefits it will offer will force you to make the transition immediately.

Lose weight

Restricting calories and increasing physical activity are widely known to result in weight loss. In addition, adopting a low-carb eating style is an excellent short-term weight loss strategy once you limit carb intake daily. When excess water in the body is managed, insulin levels drop, leading to less or no fat storage in the body.

Reverse type 2 diabetes

When the body cannot regulate blood sugar levels, diabetes occurs, affecting how the body produces and responds to insulin. Type 2 diabetes is characterized by elevated blood sugar levels that can cause kidney, eye, and nerve damage.

Following a low-carb diet drastically lowers your blood sugar levels and insulin. However, you will need guidance from your doctor before starting low-carb diets if you have been diagnosed with either type 1, type 2, or pre-diabetes.

A grateful gut

A low-carb diet is proven to manage gut problems such as irritable bowel syndrome symptoms, including cramps, pain, diarrhea, gas, and bloating. Other digestive issues like reflux and indigestion also improve.

Unfortunately, some individuals tend to believe this myth that when you take too much water, you can bloat. Contrary, bloating occurs when you consume excess carbohydrates that cause water retention in the body.

Reduce sugar cravings

Sweet foods tend to be challenging to avoid, especially when you're used to consuming them frequently or moderately. However, sugar cravings can be significantly decreased by following a low-carb, sugar-free diet.

You won't just feel full; your desire for sweets will also greatly diminish. This alone helps many people avoid sweets, facilitating weight loss and type 2 diabetes reversal. But if you really have a sweet tooth, starting low carb is just what you need to do.

Lowers the risk of heart disease

Triglycerides can sometimes be a factor in many cardiovascular issues. They are essentially little fat molecules that circulate in the blood. So, one justification for why low-carb diets lower the risk of developing cardiovascular disease is that they work to safeguard the blood vessel lining.

A higher quantity could result in accumulation in the blood vessels, which would restrict blood flow to your heart and raise your likelihood of experiencing a cardiac arrest.

Reduces risk of blood pressure

Cutting back on carbohydrates tends to lower blood pressure, which reduces your risk of developing several common ailments. Hypertension, or elevated blood pressure, poses a severe risk for various illnesses, including heart disease, renal failure, and stroke. Low-carb diets can help lower your blood pressure, which minimizes your risk of developing these diseases and lengthens your life.

Enhances brain health

Undoubtedly, all of us require carbs to maintain a healthy brain. However, a low-carb meal has the same effect. When you starve yourself or follow a low-carb plan, your brain uses the already present ketones. This has been applied for years to treat the neurological condition of epilepsy.

A low-carb diet has demonstrated incredible advantages in improving memory. It can also help those who may be at risk of having a stroke and Alzheimer's.

Reduces appetite

One of the worst side effects of dieting is hunger because it makes many individuals feel miserable, and finally, they tend to give up. But a low-carb diet results in reduced appetite with more fat and protein consumption and less calorie intake.

What to Eat On a Low Carb Diet

How to build your low-carb real food plate

According to research, one of the best approaches to losing weight is efficiently blending a low-carb diet with a low-calorie diet. Even though many low-carb foods are available, packing your plate with protein-rich, low-carb foods can help ensure that your meals are filling since they both work together to give your body the energy it requires.

Many individuals who want to reduce weight choose to eat a high-protein diet. Consuming protein makes one feel satisfied, which may cause them to reduce their calorie intake overall. But what exactly does a protein-rich, low-carb diet look like? Anything with at least the same amount of protein as net carbohydrate is acceptable.

- A low-carb diet should contain a daily limit of 20-57 grams (0.7-2 ounces) of carbs.
- Protein (0.7–0.9 grams of protein/pound (1.5–2.0 grams/kg of body weight) 40-50%
- Non-starchy vegetables (2-3 cups per day) 15-25%

- Fat (80-170 grams per day) 30-35%
- Seasoning (0.5-1.0 gram/per day)

Low-carb diets are increasingly common, but making mistakes is simple. Various obstacles can have negative consequences and produce less-than-ideal outcomes. Obesity and type 2 diabetes are two conditions that low-carb diets may help with.

However, reducing carbs alone won't help you lose weight or improve your health. The most incredible method to lose weight gradually and sustainably is by progressively adopting simple, healthy lifestyle adjustments.

Low carb meal prep tips

The best way to cut costs, reduce mealtime stress, and eat better is to prepare your meals ahead of time. Low-carb dieting might be challenging and may reduce your alternatives for eating out or taking in. Concerned that it will be challenging to maintain your low-carb diet over time? These tips will make preparing low-carb diets simple:

- Plan your meals in advance

When things get hectic, planning your meals ahead of time makes it much easier to go grocery shopping and keep your diet.

Store plenty of low-carb ingredients on hand

In this manner, you may quickly prepare a low-carb supper. For example, you may prepare a low-carb shrimp Alfredo any time if you have shirataki noodles, frozen shrimp, and Alfredo sauce.

- Prep certain foods upfront

Similarly, prepare as much as you can in advance. For example, you can prepare dressings and marinades in advance and chop vegetables and brown ground beef. Additionally, you can prepare all your meals for work the weekend before.

Having low-carb vegetables at hand will help you avoid reaching for foods that are not low-carb approved since they are a crucial part of the low-carb diet. Examples of low-carb vegetables are cauliflower, broccoli, and Brussels sprouts.

- Include frozen foods

Using frozen spinach and other vegetables on a low-carb diet can save money, minimize food waste, and streamline food preparation. Also, using frozen foods can help you reduce buying and storing fresh produce because research shows that frozen foods preserve their nutritional value quite well. However, check the labels to ensure the frozen meals you use are low in sodium and sugar, as some can be high, as the labels indicate.

- 10 ways to do a low carbohydrate diet the right way

In the current diet culture, there is a lot of misinformation about how carbs are the enemy of dieting, but that is untrue. Most diets include carbohydrates as a significant component. In reality, complex carbohydrates, which originate from whole, unrefined plant sources, are frequently packed with nutrients.

The effects on weight or blood sugar may be more significant when fewer carbohydrates are consumed. This is why we advise initially observing the nutritional guidelines quite strictly. Then, if you want to eat more carbohydrates, you can do it once you're satisfied with your health and weight.

Here are some ideas for following low-carb diets correctly, overcoming low-carb diet difficulties, and maintaining motivation as you work toward achieving your objectives.

1. Stay hydrated

One of the best things you can do for your entire body is to stay hydrated. Regular digestion can only be promoted by maintaining proper hydration. Low-carb meals can result in constipation, so it's crucial to make sure you are drinking enough water daily.

2. Eat non-starchy vegetables

Vegetables are excellent sources of fiber and minerals. Vegetables also contain phytochemicals, plant-based substances that serve as antioxidants and safeguard you from illness. However, it's crucial to concentrate on non-starchy vegetables if you are aiming to reduce your carb intake.

3. Incorporate healthy fats

For taste and aroma, potential health benefits, and satisfaction, include healthy fats in your diet plan. Your diet must have sufficient healthy fat for your body to function effectively. This is important for your physical well-being.

4. Focus on high protein

Focusing on high-protein foods is one of the best strategies to keep yourself full if you enjoy carbs but still attempting to cut back. Proteins have been proven to promote satiety, which prolongs the feeling of fullness. Thus, you might eat less during the day if you focus on more proteins.

5. Eliminate sugar-sweetened drinks

Most sugars, including glucose, sucrose, lactose, maltose, and fructose, are simple carbohydrates. Therefore, reducing your intake of sugar-sweetened drinks could help lower your chance of developing type 2 diabetes since these drinks have been linked to the start of the condition.

6. Go for whole grains

The types of carbs you pick matter a lot when making a decision. Since the entire grain is available, whole grains provide higher levels of fiber and micronutrients. The main examples are oats, millet, barley, quinoa, corn, bulgur, buckwheat, and other whole grains.

7. Check food labels for hidden sugar.

Information regarding the carbohydrate content of processed foods can be found on food labels. Watch out for some of the popular names for sugar, such as dextrose, maltose, dextrin, xylose, fructose, cane crystals, and malt syrup, on the food labels.

8. Choose low-carb snacks/breakfasts.

Even though breakfast dishes appear "healthy" at first glance, they may contain hidden levels of carbohydrates and sugar. Consider including more eggs in your morning routine if you aim for foods with less simple carbohydrates. You can feel full by including extra low-carb snacks with a substantial portion of fiber and proteins.

9. Focus quality over quantity

When treating yourself, indulge in something you like, but pay attention to the portion size. For example, if you eat a single piece of delectable cake instead of trying to stuff yourself with a fat-free, sugar-free, low-carb substitute that you don't actually like, you will probably feel more content.

10. Reconsider restaurant meals

When selecting a meal at a restaurant, pay attention to the portion sizes. When starting a low - carbohydrate diet or after choosing to drastically reduce your carb intake, eating out might be challenging. To enhance your fiber intake and make yourself feel content more quickly, consider ordering a side salad.

Low carb tips and guides

A low-carb diet may seem challenging, especially at the beginning. However, the tips below will help you stick to your diet and help you successfully experience the various benefits.

Know the different types of low-carb foods

Generally, low-carb foods include eggs, fish, nuts, chicken breast, Olive oil, pork, coconut oil, whole milk, apples, broccoli, Strawberries, and blueberries. It's also essential to have low-carb snacks between successive meals, such as cheese, hard-boiled eggs, regular carrots, and unsweetened yogurt. Don't forget to regulate the portion sizes of these snacks to avoid overeating.

Know the food serving sizes of foods and carb counts

Individuals following a low-carb diet must go for foods with a lower carbohydrate count and high nutritional value for every serving since the daily carbohydrate range for most diets is 20-50 grams. For example, 1 cup of berries, one slice of bread, half a cup of corn, one tennis ball-sized orange or apple, and 8 ounces of milk.

Meal prep

Adequate planning and meal preparation are essential in every successful low-carb diet approach. Meal prep helps save money and time and avoids unhealthy food decisions. For instance, you can prepare a week's worth of lunches or breakfasts in advance and keep them in containers for convenience.

Popular low-carb foods to prepare ahead of time include chicken lettuce wraps, egg muffins, protein pancakes, and yogurt bowls. It's important to know that all carbs are not created equal and come in different forms, such as simple and refined carbs.

If you're starting a low-carb diet, focus on reducing refined carbs for better health and weight loss results. It would help if you also considered carb cycling, which involves the consumption of low-carb foods for multiple days followed by a day of higher-carb meal consumption.

Diet diary

The perfect companion for a LC diet is a personal diary. It helps to optimize the diet and keep the goal in mind. By writing down small progress, you stay motivated. By writing down daily foods and carbohydrate intake, as well as general physical and mental well-being, you can quickly see what is working for you personally and what is not. The diet can then be adjusted and thus optimized, which in turn leads to better success.

A 14-day meal plan

Meal plans are known to make things easy. That many people find it difficult to imagine a low-carb diet, we have created a 14-day plan for you in our book. However, it should be noted that we humans are all different and therefore a diet plan should always be personalized.

At the beginning of the diet, you may feel that something is missing or that you are not really full. This may well be the case. Your body is used to carbohydrates and needs some time to adjust. By increasing your intake of healthy fats and protein, you can help your body do this. Fats are worked up differently than carbohydrates, and the body takes longer to do so, which in turn leads to a longer lasting feeling of fullness.

Planning your meals ahead of time also helps you avoid spontaneous reaches for fast food. However, don't be too hard on yourself. Sometimes you have to take a step back in order to set your sights on the goal again. With the first successes, your motivation will also increase.

14-day meal plan

14-Day Meal Plan

Week one

	Breakfast	Lunch	Dinner	Desserts
DAY 1	Sloppy Joe Sweet Potato Breakfast, Pg14	Bacon Ranch Chicken Salad Cucumber Boats, Pg28	Fluffy Omelet with Cheese and Courgette, Pg51	Keto Skillet Cookie, Pg76
DAY 2	Keto Overnight Oats, Pg15	Greek Salmon Salad, Pg29	Artichoke Chicken, Pg52	Keto Strawberry Upside-Down Cake, Pg76
DAY 3	Keto Ham and Cheese Breakfast Biscuits, Pg16	Chicken Taco Soup Recipe, Pg30	Low Carb Hamburger Stroganoff, Pg52	Keto Cucumber Avocado and Pomegranate Salad, Pg77
DAY 4	Egg Mushroom Cups, Pg16	Tuna Poke Salad, Pg30	Quick Italian Eggs, Pg53	Low Carb Blueberry Cobbler, Pg78
DAY 5	Fluffy Omelet with Cheese and Courgette, Pg17	Keto Cucumber Avocado and Pomegranate Salad, Pg32	Steak Kebabs with Chimichurri, Pg53	Easy Strawberry Banana Smoothie Bowl, Pg79
DAY 6	Breakfast Burrito Wrap with Bacon and Avocado, Pg19	Tomato Bisque with Basil Recipe, Pg32	Garlic Butter Pork Chops with Courgette, Pg54	Keto Cauliflower Wings, Pg80
DAY 7	Bacon and Spinach Egg Muffins, Pg20	Avocado Tuna Melt, Pg35	Low Carb Aubergine Pizza, Pg57	Keto No Bake Peanut Butter And Jelly Bars, Pg81

14 -Day Meal Plan

Week two

	Breakfast	Lunch	Dinner	Desserts
DAY 8	Air Fryer Avocado Baked Egg, Pg14	Chicken Club Sandwich, Pg36	Salmon in Roasted Pepper Sauce, Pg59	Keto Strawberry Upside-Down Cake, Pg76
DAY 9	Keto Breakfast Bowl, Pg22	Spicy Thai Prawns Lettuce Wraps, Pg40	Chicken Mushroom Soup, Pg69	3-ingredient No Bake Keto Peanut Butter Balls, Pg78
DAY 10	Egg Casserole Hollandaise Sauce, Pg21	Easy Keto Pizza Chaffles, Pg43	Caprese Chicken, Pg70	Easy Strawberry Banana Smoothie Bowl, Pg79
DAY 11	Keto Blueberry Pancakes, Pg23	Low Carb Steak Taco Bowl, 47	Fried Steak and Asparagus Bundles, Pg71	Keto Jalapeño Poppers, Pg83
DAY 12	Keto Ham and Cheese Breakfast Biscuits, Pg16	Pineapple Teriyaki Meatballs, Pg47	Spinach Stuffed Chicken Breasts, Pg72	Low Carb Rangoon, Pg84
DAY 13	Bacon Cauliflower Breakfast Skillet, Pg24	Vegetable Hash with Spicy Salmon Bites, Pg48	Pizza Flavored Keto Stuffed Tomato, Pg73	Low-carb Cheese Sticks, Pg84-85
DAY 14	Mango Kiwi Chia Seed Smoothie Bowl, Pg26	Coriander Lime Grilled Prawns, Pg49	Low Carb Goulash, Pg74	Easy Cheesy Courgette Breadsticks, Pg85

CHAPTER 1 BREAKFASTS

1. Sloppy Joe Sweet Potato Breakfast

Prep Time: 10 minutes | Cook Time: 30 minutes | Serves 2

- 2 sweet potatoes
- 454g minced beef
- 1 green pepper
- 1 onion
- 1 tomato
- 1 garlic clove
- 45g Worcestershire sauce
- 45g ketchup
- 14g spicy mustard
- 118ml water
- 4 eggs

Instructions

1. Put the sweet potato in a small pot and cover with cold water. Place on the stove over a high heat and bring to a boil. Cook for about 10 minutes, or until soft. Strain water and set aside.
2. While the sweet potato boils: Brown the minced beef in a sauté pan, together with the onion, green pepper and tomato.
3. Add the garlic, worcestershire sauce, ketchup, mustard, water, salt and pepper. Cover and simmer uncovered until thickened, about 20-25 minutes.
4. Optional: When the sweet potato is done, sear the cubes in a piping hot pan with some butter and season with salt and pepper.
5. Top the sweet potato with the sloppy joe and an egg fried to your liking.

Nutrition

Calories: 457 | Carbs: 25g | Protein: 27g | Fat: 27g | Sodium: 463mg | Fiber: 3g | Sugar: 10g

2. Air Fryer Avocado Baked Egg

Prep Time: 5 minutes | Cook Time: 15 minutes | Serves 2

- 1 avocado halved and seeded
- 2 small eggs
- 2g smoked paprika optional

salt and pepper to taste

Instructions

1. Preheat your Air Fryer to 390 F.
2. Cut the avocado in half and take out the seed. Using a spoon, remove some of the avocado flesh from the inside to create a larger cavity so that the egg fits in entirely.
3. Season the avocado insides with some salt and pepper, then crack the egg into the avocado.
4. Air fry the avocado with egg for about 10-15 minutes, depending on how you like the eggs.
5. Sprinkle the baked eggs with some more salt, pepper, and, if desired, smoked paprika.

Nutrition
Calories: 183 | Carbs: 6.7g | Protein: 7g | Fat: 15.2g | Sodium: 61mg | Fiber: 7g | Sugar: 1g

3. Keto Overnight Oats

Prep Time: 5 mins |Cook Time: 5 minutes | Serves 2

6g hemp heart
18g chia seeds white or black variety
200ml almond milk
20ml greek yogurt or dairy-free coconut yogurt or more almond milk
100g erythritol
0.5g cinnamon
1ml vanilla extract
7g Almond Butter
⅓ chopped dl Strawberries fresh
14g greek yogurt
0.5g coconut flakes toasted

Instructions

1. In a wide breakfast bowl, stir the hemp heart and chia seeds. Stir in any crystal sweetener at this time, if desired.
2. Stir in yogurt and milk until evenly combined. Add any vanilla or almond butter now if desired.
3. Cover the bowl tightly with plastic film wrap and refrigerate overnight. I recommend giving a good stir in the mixture 2-3 hours later to prevent the seeds from migrating to the bottom of the bowl.

4. The next day, adjust the texture by stirring in up to 3-4 tablespoons of extra unsweetened almond milk if too thick. Then, serve 1/4 of the amount as one breakfast with some fresh strawberries, toasted coconut flakes, and extra yogurt.

Nutrition

Calories: 204 |Carbs: 6.2g | Protein: 12.3g | Fat: 14.7g | Sodium: 989mg |Fiber: 3.9g | Sugar: 0.6g

4. Keto Ham and Cheese Breakfast Biscuits

Prep Time: 10 minutes | **Cook Time:** 15 minutes | **Serves** 2

- 85g cream cheese, softened
- 200g cheddar cheese
- 2 eggs
- 400g ground almonds
- 4g baking powder
- 2g salt
- 6g double cream
- 400g chopped ham
- 28g butter, melted

Instructions

1. Preheat the oven to 350 degrees.
2. In a mixing bowl combine the softened cream cheese, cheddar cheese and eggs. Stir until double cream cheese is smooth with no clumps.
3. Add ground almonds, baking powder, salt , double cream and melted butter.
4. Stir until combined.
5. Fold in the chopped ham. Do not overmix or biscuits will be tough.
6. Chill the dough for 10-15 minutes.
7. Using a small cookie or ice cream scoop, spoon the biscuits out onto a greased or lined baking sheet. Lightly press the dough down.
8. Bake for 13-15 minutes until golden. Brush with melted butter.

Nutrition

Calories: 123 |Carbs: 2.2g|Protein : 6g| Fat: 7.2g| Sodium: 48mg |Fiber: 0.3g| Sugar:3.6g

5. Egg Mushroom Cups

Prep Time: 20 minutes | Cook Time: 25 minutes | Serves 1

- 168g mushroom, whole Mushrooms

13ml Olive oil
2 extra large Egg
2g Pepper

Instructions

1. Preheat the oven to 375 degrees F.
2. Remove stem and clean out mushroom cups with a damp cloth.
3. Rub olive oil on the outside of the mushrooms.
4. Crack an egg into each cup.
5. Sprinkle with black pepper and any desired herbs, to taste.
6. Bake for 20-30 minutes until eggs are set and mushrooms are tender. Enjoy!

Nutrition

Calories: 161 | Carbs:4.3g |Protein: 8.9g | Fat: 12.4g | Sodium: 156mg|Fiber: 1.4g| Sugar: 1g

6. Fluffy Omelet with Cheese and Courgette

Prep Time: 10 minutes | Cook Time: 5 minutes | Serves 3

28g Butter
3 extra large Egg
21g Cheddar cheese
0.7g Salt
1 dash Pepper
1/2 small courgette

Instructions

1. Preheat the broiler to high temperature.
2. Heat a 10 inch (25cm) nonstick frying pan over medium heat and add butter. Once the butter sizzles, pour in egg mixture evenly over the pan. Reduce heat to low and cook until set and golden brown (about 5 minutes).
3. Remove the pan from heat and sprinkle the top of the omelet with cheese,shredded courgette, salt, and pepper. Place the omelet in a frying pan under the broiler and cook until the cheese melts, about 1-2 mins.
4. Remove the frying pan from the broiler. Gently fold the omelet in half and serve.

Nutrition

Calories: 540 | Carbs:3.4g |Protein: 27.2g| Fat: 46.4g | Sodium: 243mg |Fiber: 0.6g| Sugar: 1.6g

7. Egg-Stuffed Avocado

Prep Time: 15 minutes | Cook Time: 10 minutes | Serves 1

1 fruit, without skin and seed Avocado
2 extra large Egg
60g light mayonnaise
7.5g sour cream
2g dijon mustard
1 medium (10cm long) spring onions
1g salt

Instructions

1. Start by cooking the eggs. Fill a small saucepan 3/4 full of water. Add a good pinch of salt. This will prevent the eggs from cracking. Bring to a boil.
2. Using a spoon, dip each egg in and out of the boiling water - be careful not to get burnt. This will prevent the egg from cracking as the temperature change won't be so dramatic. After doing this a few times, carefully set the eggs in the boiling water and cook for 10 minutes. When done, remove from the heat and place in a bowl filled with cold water.
3. Peel and dice the eggs. Finely slice the spring onion.
4. In a bowl, mix the diced eggs, mayo, sour cream, Dijon mustard and most of the spring onion, leaving some for garnish. Season with salt and pepper to taste.
5. Scoop the middle of the avocado out leaving ½ - 1 inch of the avocado flesh. Cut the scooped avocado into small pieces.
6. Place the chopped avocado into the bowl with eggs and mix until well combined.
7. Fill each avocado half with the egg mixture and top with spring onion.

Nutrition

Calories: 551 | Carbs: 19.9g | Protein: 17.9g | Fat: 46.2g | Sodium: 482mg | Fiber: 9.7g

8. Meat Lovers Breakfast Pizza

Prep Time: 15 minutes | Cooking Time:15 minutes | Yield 8 slices

For the crust:
    470g shredded mozzarella
    28g cream cheese
    1 egg
    170g ground almonds
    For the topping:

6 eggs
28g double cream
14g butter
110g cooked crumbled bacon
110g cooked and crumbled breakfast sausage
110g cheese sauce
80g grated cheddar
28g chopped spring onions

Instructions

1. Preheat the oven to 425 degrees.
2. Add the mozzarella and double cream cheese to a microwave safe bowl and microwave in 20 second bursts until melted.
3. Stir to combine the cheeses and then add the egg and ground almonds.
4. Stir well to combine.
5. Place the dough on a large sheet of parchment paper. Top with a second sheet of parchment.
6. Roll the dough out into a 12 inch diameter circle.
7. Remove the top piece of parchment and transfer the bottom sheet with the dough on it to a pizza pan. Trim the parchment paper to fit the pan.
8. Bake for 10 minutes or until the crust is lightly golden.
9. Flip the crust and set aside while you prepare the eggs.
10. Whisk the eggs and double cream in a small bowl until well combined.
11. Heat a large skillet over medium heat and add the butter.
12. Once the butter has melted, add the eggs to the skillet and scramble until just slightly wet looking.
13. Top the pizza crust with the cheese sauce, followed by the eggs, bacon, and sausage. Add the cheddar over the top.
14. Return the pizza to the oven for 5 minutes.
15. Remove from the oven, sprinkle with the spring onions, slice, and serve.

Nutrition

Calories: 470|Carbs: 4g |Protein: 28g|Fat: 37g |Sodium: 840mg|Fiber: 1g| Sugar: 1g

9. Breakfast Burrito Wrap with Bacon and Avocado

Prep Time :10 minutes | Cook Time 15 minutes | Serves 1

2 eggs
30g cream

to taste salt - taste pepper
10g butter
28g mayonnaise
240ml chopped romaine lettuce
1 plum tomato
4 cooked bacon strips
½ avocado (sliced)

Instructions

1. Whisk the eggs well with the cream, salt and pepper.
2. Heat up a non-stick pan to a medium heat.
3. Melt half the butter in the pan, and pour in half the egg mixture. Immediately tilt the pan back and forth to ensure the egg covers the entire base.
4. Cover the pan and let the cook for about a minute.
5. When you are able to move the entire crepe when shaking the pan back and forth, carefully flip it over with a spatula.
6. When it's fully cooked, transfer to a paper towel to remove excess oiliness.
7. Repeat with the other half of the egg mix.
8. Spread the mayonnaise on the crepe.
9. Add the lettuce, tomato, bacon and avocado.
10. Season with salt and pepper.
11. Roll and enjoy!

Nutrition

Calories: 410| Carbs: 7g | Protein: 13g | Fat: 37g | Sodium: 473mg | Fiber: 4g | Sugar: 2g

10. Bacon and Spinach Egg Muffins

Prep Time: 15 minutes | Cook Time: 15 minutes | Serves 12

12 large eggs
12 slices sugar free bacon
250g baby spinach ¼ cup diced onion any kind
59ml unsweetened almond milk
5ml avocado oil
1g salt
6g pepper

Instructions

1. Preheat your oven to 375°F (190°C). While it preheats, cook the bacon in a large skillet over medium heat until it's nice and crispy. Set it aside on a paper towel lined plate to cool.
2. Dice the onion and spinach. Once the bacon is cooled enough to handle, cut it into bitesized pieces.
3. Crack the eggs into a large bowl. Add the milk, salt, and pepper. Whisk it all together until fully combined.
4. Spray or drizzle a muffin tin well with oil. Add the spinach, onion, and bacon in each well, then pour the egg mixture on top, until each is filled to about 80%.
5. Bake for 18-22 minutes, or until the eggs are cooked through.

Nutrition
Calories: 127 | Carbs: 1g | Protein: 8g | Fat: 10g | Sodium: 193mg | Fiber: 1g | Sugar: 1g

11. Egg Casserole Hollandaise Sauce

Prep Time 10 minutes | Cook Time: 30-35 minutes | Serves 10-12

   12 eggs beaten
   29ml canned coconut milk, unsweetened
   14ml olive oil
   64g chopped yellow onion
   6 asparagus spears, chopped into 1 inch chunks
   6 slices cooked bacon, chopped (divided)
   2 garlic cloves, minced
   Salt and pepper to taste
Hollandaise Sauce
   118ml melted ghee
   4ml Franks Hot Sauce
   2.84g salt
   3 large egg yolks
   14.7 ml lemon juice
   1.4g cayenne pepper

Instructions

Egg Casserole
   1 Preheat the oven to 350F. Spray a 8X8 OR 9X13" baking dish.
   2 Heat a medium skillet over medium-high heat with olive oil.
   3 Add the minced garlic, chopped onion, 3 slices bacon, chopped and asparagus chunks to the skillet.

4 Sauté together for around 4-5 minutes or until tender

5 Meanwhile, in a large mixing bowl, whisk together the eggs and coconut milk and season very liberally with salt and black pepper (about 1 tsp salt and 3/4 tsp black pepper)

6 Transfer the sauteéd veggies into the beaten eggs and whisk together until combined.

7 Pour the mixture into the 9X13" baking dish.

8 Bake for 30-35 minutes.

9 About 10 minutes before the casserole is finished cooking, make the hollandaise sauce below.

10 Remove the casserole from the oven and let it cool for 5 minutes.

11 Pour the hollandaise sauce over the entire casserole and top with the remaining chopped bacon.

12 Enjoy!

Hollandaise Sauce

1 Add 3 egg yolks, lemon juice, salt, hot sauce and cayenne pepper to a mason jar.

2 Heat 118ml ghee over low heat until completely melted.

3 Add a little bit of the melted to the mason jar and use an on immersion blender at high speed to start blending together. Slowly pour the rest of the melted ghee in the jar as you are blending. As you blend, the sauce will begin to thicken.

Nutrition

Calories: 260 |Carbs: 5g|Protein: 13g | Sodium: 300g |Fat: 22g | Fiber: 2g |Sugar: 2g

12. Keto Breakfast Bowl

Prep Time: 5 minutes | Cook Time: 25 minutes | Serves 2

142g greens
1 clove garlic crushed
15ml olive oil
250g bell peppers
227g breakfast sausage
6 eggs
30g double cream

Instructions

1. Heat up a large nonstick skillet to medium heat and then add 2 teaspoons of olive oil and the crushed garlic. Saute for a minute and then add the greens. Start with a big handful and keep mixing to wilt and shrink the greens. Keep adding more until all the greens are done. You can season with salt and black pepper if you wish. Take the greens out of the pan and set aside.

2. Using the same pan, again heat to medium heat and add the remaining 1 teaspoon of olive oil and then the bell peppers. Saute until softened which should take about 4-5 minutes. When done take out of the pan and set aside.

3. Using the same pan, spray with nonstick cooking spray and heat to medium heat. In a blender add the eggs and double cream and blend until well combined. Pour into the preheated pan and cook as you would scrambled eggs. Use a silicone spatula to push the outside toward the middle until you get all the eggs cooked then take out of the pan and set aside.

4. Lastly use the same pan for the last time and spray again with the cooking spray. Brown sausage until there is no pink showing and it's cooked through.

Nutrition
Calories: 506 | Carbs: 12.2g | Protein: 27.8g | Fat: 39g | Sodium: 715mg | Fiber: 2.9g | Sugar: 6.1g

13. Keto Blueberry Pancakes

Prep Time: 10 minutes | Cook Time: 20 minutes | 10 Pancakes

Pancake Ingredients
57g softened cream cheese
2 eggs
38g ground almonds
12g Swerve brown sugar
31g cream
1 ml vanilla extract
Pinch salt
Blueberry Syrup Ingredients
83g fresh blueberries
75g Swerve or similar low carb sweetener
15ml water

Instructions
Blueberry Syrup
1. In a microwave safe bowl, combine ¾ cup blueberries, sugar and water. Mix well and microwave for 1-2 minutes.
2. Add remaining blueberries to sauce and allow to cool for 20 minutes.

Pancakes
1. Combine all pancake ingredients using a blender.
2. Grease a flat-griddle or non-stick pan over medium heat. Pour a scoop of batter onto the pan. Flip when bubbles start to form on the surface. Repeat until all batter is used.

3. Stack pancakes and top with blueberry syrup.
Nutrition
Calories: 88 | Carbs: 4g| Protein: 3g| Fat: 6.60g| Sodium: 280mg | Fiber: 0.6g|Sugar:4g

14. Chia seed porridge

Prep Time: 10 minutes | Cook Time: 15 minutes | Serves 2

20g erythritol or other sugar substitute.
60g chia seeds
40 g coconut flour
300ml water
200ml almond milk
8g coconut shreds

Preparation.
1.Mix the chia seeds with 2 tablespoons each of almond milk and water in a small bowl and let them steep briefly.
2.Meanwhile, in a saucepan over medium heat, heat the coconut flour with the remaining almond milk and water.
3. Add the erythritol, chia seeds and coconut flakes, stirring constantly. Cook briefly until the coconut flour thickens the porridge slightly.
If you like it creamier, add a little more almond milk. For a little extra, you can sprinkle chopped nuts over the porridge.
4.Enjoy hot.

Healthy chia seeds instead of oatmeal, almond milk and shredded coconut make this porridge especially tasty.

Nutrition
Calories: 281 |Carbs: 16g| Protein: 1 2g| Fat: 19g| Sodium: 2704mg| Fiber: 0.3g | Sugar:5g

15. Bacon Cauliflower Breakfast Skillet

Prep Time:10 minutes | Cook Time: 15 minutes | Serves 2

400g cauliflower
½ diced onion
½ diced red bell pepper
4 bacon strips cut into bite-sized pieces
4 eggs boiled - your preferences we boiled ours for 8 minutes to medium hard

119g double cream
1g paprika
14g butter to taste
salt and pepper to taste

Instructions
1. Sauté the bacon and onion together until the bacon is cooked and the onion is soft.
2. Add the cauliflower, red bell pepper, paprika, butter and season with salt and pepper.
3. Sauté everything together until the cauliflower is cooked to your liking [about 5-10 minutes]
4. Add the double cream and stir until everything is hot and blended.
5. Add the boiled eggs on top and garnish with fresh parsley. Serve hot and enjoy!

Nutrition
Calories: 677 | Carbs: 18.7g | Protein 32.6g| Fat: 53.6g | Sodium: 1105mg| Fiber: 6.2g| Sugar: 8.8g

16. Keto Bacon and Egg Breakfast Bowls

Prep Time: 15 minutes | Cook Time: 15 minutes | Serves 2

¾ bag frozen cauliflower rice
¼ chopped onion
3 strips bacon
2 large eggs
2g salt
2g coarse black pepper
10g butter

Instructions
1. Cut strips of bacon into pieces and slice onion up as well. Place frozen cauliflower rice bags in the microwave and drain excess water when it's finished.
2. With pan on medium high heat begin to crisp bacon and after the bacon has released some fat into the pan toss in onions to caramelize
3. Lower heat if the pan starts to get too hot you don't want to burn the bacon or onions.
4. Once bacon and onions have a great color to them, toss in cauliflower rice. Season with salt and pepper. Then toss butter on top and continue to mix everything together.
5. Cauliflower rice will absorb all the bacon fat in the pan so no need to drain. Cook for about 3-5 minutes and remove from heat.

6. Scramble or fry your eggs however you like and top the dish off with them. Sunny side up seemed to work the best but scrambled is always super easy.

Nutrition
Calories: 27 |Carbs: 2.3g|Protein: 17.1g |Fat: 21.2g | Sodium: 1051mg | Fiber: 0.4g | Sugar: 1g

17. Low-Carb Sweet Potato Breakfast with Poached Egg

Prep Time: 10 minutes | Cook Time: 10 minutes | Serves 4

2 Sweet Potatoes, shredded
4 eggs
8 bacon strips, chopped
to taste salt and pepper
113g fresh basil, chopped
14g olive loil

Instructions
1. Cook the sweet potato in the oil over medium-high heat for approximately 10 minutes, until cooked. Season with salt and pepper to taste.
2. While the sweet potato cooks, bring a shallow saucepan filled with water to the boil. Once boiling, bring down to a light simmer. Crack the eggs into the simmering water and let cook for 2-3 minutes for a soft egg. Remove with a slotted spoon.
3. Divide the sweet potato hash into plates, top each with an egg, chopped bacon and fresh basil.

Nutrition
Calories: 305 | Carbs: 14g | Protein: 12g | Fat: 22g | Sodium: 390mg | Fiber: 2g | Sugar: 3g

18. Mango Kiwi Chia Seed Smoothie Bowl

Prep Time: 5 minutes | Cook Time: 10 minutes | Serves 2

24g chia seeds
355ml unsweetened almond milk
2 medium bananas sliced and frozen
400g frozen mango chunks
2 kiwis peeled and sliced optional toppings

24g chia seeds

Instructions

1. In a small bowl, add chia seeds and 64g almond milk. Give it a good whisk, until thoroughly combined. Cover and let set in the fridge for about 10 minutes.
2. Add bananas and the remaining 250g almond milk to a blender. Blend until smooth, scraping down the sides of the blender as need. Add mangoes, blending until mostly smooth.
3. Take the chia seed mixture out of the fridge—it should have thickened to a gel-like consistency. Give it another good whisk. Using a rubber spatula or spoon, scrape the chia seed mixture out of the cup and into the blender. Blend until smooth.
4. Pour into two bowls. Top with kiwi slices. Add additional toppings as you'd like. Enjoy!

Nutrition

Calories 285 | Carbs: 64.7g | Protein 4.4g | Fat: 5g | Fiber: 9.1g | Sodium: 140mg | Sugar: 43.8g

CHAPTER 2 LUNCH

1. Bacon Ranch ChickenSalad Cucumber Boats

Prep Time: 10 minutes | Cook Time: 5 minutes | Yield: 8 cucumber boats

10ml avocado oil
425g canned chicken

6g dried dill
1g dried parsley
2g garlic powder
2g onion powder
2g pepper
1g salt
84g sour cream
64g shredded sharp cheddar cheese
150g crumbled cooked bacon
5ml apple cider vinegar
4 cucumbers recommended that they be chilled in the refrigerator
Flakey sea salt
Freshly - cracked pepper

Instructions

1. In a pan over medium heat, heat oil until glistening. Add canned chicken and cook for about 1 minute. Add spices and cook until spices are fragrant, about 1-2 minutes. Transfer chicken to a mixing bowl and add sour cream. Mix ingredients until well-combined. Add shredded cheddar, crumbled bacon, and apple cider vinegar and mix again.
2. Cover bowl with lid or foil and transfer to refrigerator to chill for 15 minutes.
3. While chicken salad chills, prepare cucumber boats by cutting cucumbers in half lengthwise, removing seeds with a spoon, and blotting dry with a paper towel.
4. Remove chilled chicken salad from the refrigerator and spoon into the cucumber boats. Sprinkle flakey sea salt and crack pepper atop cucumber boats then serve.

Nutrition

Calories: 265| Carbs:7.3g|Protein: 25.9g |Fat: 14.7g |Sodium: 637mg | Fiber:1g | Sugar: 2.7g

2. Greek Salmon Salad

Prep Time: 20 minute | Cook Time: 15 minutes | Serves 4

Salmon:
  4 salmon fillets room temperature
  Coarse sea salt and pepper to taste
  16ml olive oil
  1 lemon
Greek Salad:
  330g cherry tomatoes

400g English cucumbers chopped into pieces
   64g red onion
   113g feta
Greek Vinaigrette:
   59ml olive oil
   30ml red wine vinegar
   1 clove garlic minced
   3g dried oregano
   3g dijon mustard
   3g salt and 1.5g pepper

Instructions

1. Pat the salmon dry with a paper towel and season with salt and pepper. In a large nonstick skillet, heat the olive oil over medium-high heat. Add the salmon to the pan and press down making sure the fillets have full contact with the pan. Let them cook 3-4 minutes without disturbing them until they get a golden brown crust. Flip them over and cook for 2-3 minutes or until desired doneness. Salmon should flake easily with a fork. Remove from the pan and squeeze lemon over the top.
2. While the salmon is cooking, prepare the Greek vinaigrette. Whisk together all the vinaigrette ingredients in a small bowl and set aside.
3. In a medium bowl, add the tomatoes, cucumbers, and red onion. Drizzle the vinaigrette over the veggies and toss to coat. Gently stir in the feta.
4. To assemble the salad: Place a handful of lettuce on each plate and top with the Greek veggies tossed in the vinaigrette. Place your salmon on top. Add a squeeze of lemon and enjoy. Salmon can be eat warm, room temperature, or cold depending on your preference.

Nutrition

Calories: 595 | Carbs: 10.1g | Protein: 46.3g |Fat: 42.3g | Sodium: 529mg |Fiber: 3.1g| Sugar:5.5g

3. Chicken Taco Soup Recipe

Prep Time: 20minutes | Cook Time: 45minutes | Serves 2

   500g chicken breast
   14ml olive oil
   1 diced onion
   2 diced celery stalks
   400g diced tomatoes
   2 diced jalapeno pepper seeds removed and finely

4g dried oregano
4g ground cumin
2g paprika
1892ml chicken stock
1 lime juice
64g fresh coriander
to taste salt and pepper
to taste sour cream
to taste avocado

Instructions

1. Start by sautéing the onion and celery in oil, in a large pot until soft, about 10 minutes.
2. Chuck everything else in the pot [except coriander], bring to a boil and then allow to simmer for 45 minutes.
3. After 45 minutes, remove the chicken and shred it up with two forks! Throw it back in the pot, along with the fresh coriander.
4. Do a little taste test and add salt/pepper if needed.
5. Serve up the soup with a generous dollop of sour cream. Fresh avocado on the side makes it extra delicious!

Nutrition

Calories: 88.6 | Carbs: 8g | Protein: 8.2g | Fat: 3.3g | Sodium: 905.9mg | Fiber: 1.79g | Sugar: 3.4g

4. Tuna Poke Salad

Prep Time: 15 minutes | Cook Time: 0 minutes | Serves 2

227g sushi grade tuna
32g sliced spring onions
29ml reduced sodium soy sauce
5ml sesame oil
2.5ml sriracha
15 ml less sodium soy sauce
6g wasabi
30ml rice wine vinegar
7ml sesame oil
85g baby greens
250g cucumbers
1 small Hass avocado sliced
64g shelled edamame

Instructions

1. Combine the vinaigrette ingredients in a small bowl and set aside.
2. In a medium bowl, combine tuna with spring onions, soy sauce, sesame oil and sriracha. Gently toss to combine and set aside while you prepare the salad.
3. In 2 bowls, layer the salad greens, 1/2 of the tuna, edamame, avocado, cucumber and drizzle with Soy-Wasabi Vinaigrette.
4. Top with furikake and spring onions, for garnish.

Nutrition

Calories: 404 |Carbs:16g | Protein: 36g |Fat: 23g | Sodium: 1211.5mg|Fiber: 7.5g| Sugar: 3.5g

5. Rocket Salad with Crispy Prosciutto

Prep Time: 35 minutes | Cook Time: 35 minutes | Serves 2

- 57g sliced prosciutto
- 1182g baby rocket
- 32g shaved parmesan cheese
- olive oil spray
- 2 large eggs fresh black pepper
- 28g minced shallots
- 30ml extra virgin olive oil
- 15ml sherry vinegar
- 10ml Dijon mustard
- 2g honey

Instructions

1. Preheat the oven to 375°F. Line a large baking sheet with parchment paper.
2. Arrange the prosciutto on the prepared baking sheet and bake for 15 minutes or until lightly browned and crisp. Crumble into large pieces.
3. Meanwhile, whisk the dressing ingredients in a large bowl. Add the rocket and toss well. Divide on two plates and top with crumbled prosciutto and parmesan.
4. To cook the eggs heat a large nonstick skillet over medium-low heat, spray with oil and gently break the eggs. Season with salt and cook, covered until the whites are set and the yolks are still runny, or longer if desired. Place the egg on top of each salad and serve with fresh pepper, if desired.

Nutrition

Calories: 344 |Carbs: 8g |Protein: 18.5g | Fat:24g | Sodium: 1043mg| Fiber: 1.5g| Sugar: 4g

6. Easy Braised Chicken Drumsticks in Tomatillo Sauce

Prep Time:10 minutes | Cook Time: 30 minutes | Serves 6

- 6 chicken drumsticks
- 15ml cider vinegar
- 5g coarse sea salt
- 6g black pepper
- 6g dried oregano
- 5ml olive oil
- 64g jarred tomatillo sauce
- 32g chopped coriander
- 1 jalapeno

Instructions

1. Season chicken with vinegar, salt, pepper and oregano. Marinate a few hours if time permits.
2. Set the Instant Pot to saute, when hot add the oil and the chicken to brown on both sides, about 4 minutes on each side.
3. Add the tomatillo salsa, the 32g chopped coriander and jalapeno, cover and cook on high pressure for 20 minutes, until the chicken is tender. When the pressure releases, garnish with coriander and serve over rice if desired.
4. Place ingredients in the slow cooker and cook low 6 hours or high 3 hours.
5. Follow same directions, add a little water and cook covered on low until chicken is very tender, 30 to 40 minutes

Nutrition
Calories: 161| Carbs: 5g | Protein: 22g | Fat: 5g |Sodium: 736mg |Fiber: 7g | Sugar: 2g

7. Tomato Bisque with Basil Recipe

Prep Time: 15 minutes | Cook Time: 45 minutes | Serves 4

- 2 cans diced tomatoes
- 1 onion, diced
- 2 celery stalks, diced
- 2 cloves garlic, minced
- 14g tomato paste
- 8g dried basil
- 1419ml vegetable stock
- Salt and pepper to taste

118ml double cream

Instructions

1. Sauté the onion and celery in a medium sized pot until soft [about 5 minutes].
2. Add all the rest of the ingredients [except the cream] and allow to simmer for 45 minutes.
3. Use an immersion blender, and blend until smooth.
4. Now, stir in the cream.
5. Garnish with fresh basil and serve immediately.

Nutrition

Calories: 173 | Carbs: 18g | Protein: 3g | Fat: 11g | Sodium: 1477mg | Fiber: 3g | Sugar: 10g

8. Chicken Broccoli Salad

Prep Time: 15 minutes | Total Time: 15 minutes | Serves 6

950g chopped Broccoli
75g chopped Red Onion
340g Cooked Chicken
7 strips Bacon cooked and crumbled
75g Mayo
110g Greek Yogurt plain unsweetened
3g Garlic Salt
30ml Lemon juice

Instructions

1. In a large bowl, combine chopped broccoli, chopped red onion and chicken.
2. In a separate bowl, whisk together mayo, greek yogurt, and garlic salt.
3. Pour the dressing over the chopped ingredients and mix well.
4. Stir in lemon juice and 5 crumbed strips of bacon.
5. Add salt and pepper to taste.
6. When you are ready to serve, garnish with remaining bacon crumbles.

Nutrition

Calories: 275 | Carbs: 9.9g | Protein: 28.3g | Fat: 12.2g | Sodium: 602mg | Fiber: 3.7g | Sugar: 0g

9. Quick Buffalo Chicken Salad

Prep Time: 15 minutes | Total Time: 15 minutes | Serves 1

14g pepper or hot sauce
51g canned chicken
15g spinach
1/2 medium tomatoes

Instructions

1. Mix hot sauce with chicken. Put on top of spinach, and add tomatoes to top. Toss together and enjoy!

Nutrition

Calories: 228 | Carbs: 8.8g | Protein: 28.4g | Fat: 8.8g | Sodium: 57mg | Fiber: 2.1g | Sugar: 3g

10. Black Bean Avocado Salad

Prep Time: 15 minutes | Total Time: 15 minutes | Serves 4

2 cans of black beans
1 can of corn kernels
3–4 ripe avocados
2 jalapeños (optional or sub bell pepper)
130g coriander
1 medium red onion
210g cherry tomatoes
4-5 lemons, juiced
Salt and pepper to taste

Instructions

1. Dice the onion, cut the cherry tomatoes in half and chop the coriander. Open cans of beans and corn, drain and rinse.
2. Cut the avocados last so they don't brown.
3. Add everything to a large mixing bowl along with the lemon juice, salt, and pepper.
4. Taste and add salt, pepper, lime juice as needed. Serve with tortilla chips, tostadas or eaten with a spoon!

Nutrition

Calories: 230 | Carbs: 25.3g | Protein: 5.8g | Fat: 14.1g | Sodium: 20mg | Fiber: 10g | Sugar: 7g

11. Citrus Prawns and Avocado Salad

Prep Time: 15 minutes | Cook Time: 45 minutes | Serves 4

454g medium Pan-Seared Citrus Prawns
128g greens
30ml extra virgin olive oil
Juice of 1/2 lemon or 1/2 orange
1 diced avocado sliced or
1 shallot minced
113g sliced almonds
Coarse sea salt and freshly ground black pepper

Instructions

1. Prepare the recipe for the Pan-Seared Citrus Prawns, or gently warm the leftover prawns. Or, if you prefer, serve the prawns chilled.
2. Toss the prawns with the salad greens in a large bowl.
3. Lightly drizzle with olive oil, and if desired, some of the sauce remaining from the prawns with a generous squeeze of citrus, and toss lightly to coat.
4. Add the avocado, shallots and sliced almonds and then season with coarse sea salt and freshly ground black pepper and serve

Nutrition

Calories: 374 | Carbs: 14g | Protein: 31g|Fat: 23g |Sodium: 906mg|Fiber: 7g | Sugar: 2g

12. Avocado Tuna Melt

Prep Time: 10 minutes | Cook Time: 10 minutes | Serves 4

2 avocado
1 can tuna
32g onion
32g pickles
32g red bell pepper
2g paprika
58g mayonnaise
64g cheddar cheese
to taste salt and pepper

Instructions

1. Preheat the oven to 400°F/200°C.
2. Scoop out some of the avocado to make to hole slightly bigger. Mix the bit of scooped out avocado into the tuna salad.

3. Mix the tuna, onion, red bell pepper, pickle, cheese, paprika and mayo. Season to your liking with salt and pepper.
4. Scoop the tuna mixture into the avocado and top with more cheese.
5. Slide into the oven for approximately 5-10 minutes. Until the cheese is melted.

Nutrition

Calories: 359 |Carbs: 11g |Protein: 14g|Fat: 30g| Sodium: 368mg| Fiber: 7g |Sugar: 2g

13. Green Bean Salad

Prep Time: 10 minutes | Cook Time: 10 minutes | Serves 2

- 64g green beans
- 64g can sliced black olives
- 44ml balsamic vinegar
- 44ml extra virgin olive oil
- 3 chopped medium spring onions
- 4g coarse sea salt
- fresh black pepper to taste
- 5 hard boiled eggs peeled and sliced

Instructions

1. Place green beans in a large pot and cover with water, about 6 cups. Bring to a boil, then cover and cook until tender crisp, about 6 minutes
2. Drain and rinse under cold water when done to prevent them from overcooking, drain.
3. In a large bowl, combine balsamic, oil, salt and pepper. Toss in the green beans, spring onions and olives.
4. Mix well and top with sliced eggs. Refrigerate and serve chilled or room temperature.

Nutrition

Calories: 176 | Carbs: 11g | Protein: 7.5g| Fat: 12g | Sodium: 308mg |Fiber: 4.5g | Sugar: 4g

14. Chicken Club Sandwich

Prep Time: 10 minutes | Cook Time: 10 minutes | Serves 2

- 6 Lettuce Leaves Iceberg
- 170g Chicken Breast cooked
- 4 Slices of Bacon
- 113g Deli Ham

2 Slices Cheese
4 Slices Tomatoes
15g Mayo

Instructions

1. Cook the bacon and warm up the cooked chicken. Separate the lettuce leaves into "sandwich bread" sizes.
2. Lay 2 lettuce leaves onto a plate and spread 1/2 of the may on the lettuce. Next layer the ham, chicken and cheese on top. Cover the meat with the other 2 lettuce leaves and spread the other 1/2 of the mayo on top of them.
3. Place the tomato slices and bacon on top of that. Cover with the last two lettuce slices. Slice the sandwich into 4, by slicing corner to corner.
4. This recipe makes 2 servings or 4 small sandwiches.

Nutrition
Calories: 400 | Carbs: 6.2g | Protein: 39g| Fat: 24.3g |Sodium : 1548mg | Fiber: 0.9g

15. Stuffed Sweet Potatoes

Prep Time:15minutes | Cook Time: 1 hr | Serves 4

4 sweet potatoes
250g button mushrooms
250g cheddar cheese
250g bacon
64g chicken stock
236ml doule cream
8g dried chives
8gdried thyme
Salt and pepper to taste
5g spring onions

Instructions

1. Preheat the oven 400°F/200°C.
2. Coat the sweet potatoes with olive oil and salt and bake on a baking sheet, uncovered for
45-60 minutes. Until it pierces easily with a knife.
3. While the potatoes cook, sauté the bacon and mushrooms in a pan until crisp.
4. Add the doule cream and cheese and cook until the cheese is melted and the sauce thickens.Season with salt and pepper if needed to own taste.
5. Once the sweet potatoes are ready, cut them in half lengthwise and scoop some of the flesh out, to create a boat.

6. Spoon some of the sauce into each of the boats, garnish with chopped spring onions and serve immediately.

Nutrition

Calories: 477 | Carbs: 31g |Protein: 13g | Fat: 35g | Sodium: 534mg |Fiber: 5g | Sugar:6g

16. Low-Carb & Keto Greek Chicken Bowls

Prep Time:15 minutes | Cook Time:10 minutes | Serves 4

Greek Chicken
- 450g boneless chicken
- 44ml olive oil
- 30ml lemon juice
- 15ml red wine vinegar
- 14g Greek seasoning
- 0.5g sea salt

Tzatziki Sauce
- 230g full-fat plain Greek yogurt
- ½ grated medium Persian cucumber
- 2 grated cloves garlic
- Zest of 1 medium lemon
- 15ml fresh lemon juice
- 28g minced fresh dill
- Sea salt, as needed

Red Wine Vinegar Dressing
- Black pepper, as needed
- 44ml olive oil
- 15ml red wine vinegar
- 4g minced fresh oregano
- Sea salt, to taste

Salad Toppings
- 1 diced large cucumber
- 200g cherry tomatoes halved
- 100g thinly sliced red onion
- 80g pitted Kalamata olives
- 110g feta cheese

Instructions

1. To make the chicken, combine the chicken, oil, lemon juice, vinegar, Greek seasoning, and salt in a sealable container. Marinate the chicken in the refrigerator for 30 minutes or up to overnight.
2. To make the tzatziki, stir together the yogurt, cucumber, garlic, lemon zest, lemon juice, dill, salt, and black pepper in a medium bowl. Refrigerate the tzatziki until you are ready to serve.
3. Heat a 10-inch (25-cm) or larger cast-iron skillet over medium-high heat. Add the chicken and marinade to the skillet. Cook the chicken for 3 to 4 minutes per side, until it is brown and its internal temperature reaches 165°F (74°C).
4. To make the red wine vinegar dressing, whisk together the oil, vinegar, oregano, and salt in a small bowl.
5. To assemble the bowls, divide the chicken among four individual serving bowls. Top the chicken with the cucumber, tomatoes, onion, olives, and feta cheese. Pour the red wine vinegar dressing over the bowls and top each bowl with the tzatziki just before serving.

Nutrition
Calories: 496 |Carbs: 12.6g |Protein: 40.4g |Fat: 32.3g | Sodium: 1023mg |Fiber: 2.3g

17. Thai Chicken Lettuce Wraps

Prep Time: 5 minutes | Cook Time: 10 minutes | Serves 6

15 ml sesame oil
32g diced onion
2 cloves of garlic
14ml fresh minced ginger or ginger paste
284g minced chicken
59ml Tamari or soy sauce
14ml Thai sweet red chili sauce
juice of 1 lime
6g maple syrup or honey
37g chopped cashews
32g chopped spring onions
32g chopped coriander fresh
32g carrots shredded Sesame seeds for topping
1 head butter lettuce - leaves removed rinsed and dried

Instructions

1. Make the garlic, ginger pan sauce. Heat up a pan to medium high heat and add the oil. Once the oil is hot, add in the onions. Toss and let cook for 2-3 minutes until the onions start to brown and turn translucent. Then add in the garlic and ginger. Toss that all together and let it cook for 2 minutes.
2. Cook the chicken. Add the minced chicken to the pan, tossing it in the pan sauce while breaking it up with a wooden spoon or spatula. Season the chicken with a little salt and pepper and let it cook until it starts to turn golden brown and there is no more pink, about 3-4 minutes.
3. Make the thai chili sauce. Meanwhile, add the soy sauce, chili sauce, lime juice, and honey to a small bowl and mix to combine.
4. Add the sauce to the chicken. Sprinkle the chopped cashews over the chicken in the pan and pour in the sauce. Toss that all together, reduce the heat to low and let that all cook for 2 more minutes. Remove the pan from the heat and let it cool for a few minutes, then stir in the carrots, chopped spring onions and coriander.
5. Assemble the lettuce wraps. To assemble the lettuce wraps, open one of the lettuce leaves and add a large spoonful of the chicken mixture into the wrap and top it with some of the pan sauce and sesame seeds. Continue until you have made all of the lettuce wraps.

Nutrition
Calories: 158| Carbs: 8g |Fat: 9g | Sodium: 631mg | Protein: 11g | Fiber: 1g | Sugar: 5g

18. Spicy Thai Prawns Lettuce Wraps

Prep Time: 10 minutes | Cook Time: 4 minutes | Marinating 30 minutes | Serves 4

Thai Prawns:
    454g prawns
    10g coconut aminos
    59ml olive oil
    14ml fish sauce
    10ml lime juice
    1g crushed red pepper flakes
Lettuce Wraps:
    16 leaves butterhead lettuce
    ⅓ small cucumber
    1 large avocado
Peanut Sause:
    67g peanut butter

20g coconut aminos
22ml lime juice
2g crushed red pepper flakes
½g sea salt
1g garlic powder
Optional garnishes
Spring onionsPeanuts
Lime wedges

Instructions

1. In a medium bowl, whisk together the coconut aminos, 30 ml olive oil, fish sauce, lime juice, and crushed red peppers.
2. Add the prawns and mix to coat. Cover and let sit for 30 minutes to marinate.
3. Meanwhile, whisk together the ingredients for the peanut sauce. Set aside.
4. Heat the remaining 2 tablespoons (30mL) oil in a large pan or wok over medium heat. Add the prawns and saute for 4-6 minutes, until white, opaque, and cooked through.
5. Divide the prawns, cucumbers, and avocados among the lettuce leaves. Drizzle with peanut sauce. If desired, garnish with spring onions, roasted peanuts, and lime wedges.

Nutrition

Calories: 470 | Carbs: 16g |Fat: 31g |Sodium: 783mg |Protein: 29g |Fiber: 6g|Sugar:8g

19.Carne Asada Salad

Prep Time: 10 minutes | Cook Time: 10 minutes | Serves 2

1 beef Strip Steak Boneless
1 large clove garlic
4g ground cumin
2g coarse sea salt and black pepper to taste
360g mixed greens
64g pico de gallo
32g shredded Monterrey Jack
2 lime wedges
64g prepared or my homemade guacamole
Additional lime wedges
jalapeno slices

Instructions

1. Rub garlic all over the meat then season with salt, cumin and black pepper.

2. To broil, place steak on a rack in a broiler pan so the surface of beef is 3 to 4 inches from heat. Broil about 3 minutes on each side for medium rare to medium. To grill, heat the grill and oil the grates. When hot, grill over medium-high heat about 3 minutes on each side for medium rare to medium. To cook in a skillet, Heat a skillet over high heat and let the skillet get very hot. When it's hot, spray with oil and cook the steaks for about 3 minutes on each side for medium rare to medium.
3. Squeeze juice from 1 lime wedge over each steak. Slice Steaks into thin slices.
4. To serve, divide the lettuce, pico de gallo, cheese and guacamole between two plates.
5. Serve with steak; garnish with lime wedges and jalapeño, if desired.

Nutrition
Calories: 390 Carbs: 12g | Protein: 38g | Fat: 21.5g |Sodium: 542.5mg |Fiber: 6.5g | Sugar: 1g

20.Pan-Seared Filet Mignon Recipe with Herb Butter

Prep Time: 10 minutes | Cook Time: 10 minutes | Serves 4

4 (280g) thick tenderloin beef filets (roughly 2 inches thick)
28g butter
salt and pepper to taste
1/2 stick of butter
14g chopped fresh rosemary
14g chopped fresh tarragon
7g minced garlic

Instructions
1. Soften the butter in a microwave safe bowl until malleable, 10-15 seconds.
2. Stir in herbs and garlic until fully mixed. Spoon the butter onto tin foil doing your best to reshape it to resemble a stick of butter.
3. Place in the refrigerator for about 10 minutes and remove 5 minutes before adding to the filet.

For The Filefts
1. Preheat the oven to 415° F. Remove steak from the fridge 30 minutes before cooking, this is to bring the steak to room temperature and ensureyour cooking times are more accurate. Season both sides generously with salt and pepper.
2. Add the plain butter to an oven safe cast iron skillet and turn up high,allow the skillet to become scorching hot first. Place the filets face down and sear undisturbed for 2 minutes. Flip the filets and sear for an additional 2 minutes. This will give your filets a nice seared edge.

3. Transfer your skillet directly to the oven. For rare, bake for 4 minutes. Medium rare, 5-6 minutes. Medium, 6-7 minutes. Medium well, 8-9 minutes. Remember, depending on the size of the steak, the more or less time itwill take. This recipe is ideal for a 224g -280g portion, roughly 2-3 inchesthick.
4. Remove filets from the skillet and set on a plate, lightly cover with tin foil and let sit for 5 minutes before serving. This is important to bring your steak to its final serving temperature.
5. Top with a slice of garlic and herb butter and serve.

Nutrition

Calories: 858 |Carbs: 1.1g |Protein: 55.4g |Fat: 67.5g |Sodium: 552mg| Fiber:0.4g | Sugar: 0g

21. Cheesy Taco Minced Beef & Cauliflower Rice Skillet

Prep Time: 5 minutes | Cook Time: 25 minutes | Serves 6

450g minced beef
1 (570g) bag frozen cauliflower rice
1 (280g) can diced tomatoes & chilies
1 packet taco seasoning
100ml water
1 diced bell pepper
1 small diced yellow onion
14ml oil
100g cheddar cheese

Instructions

1. In a large pan set to medium heat, sauté the diced onion and bell pepper with about a tbsp of oil for 3-4 minutes or until they start to become soft.
2. Add the minced beef to the pan and cook until no longer pink; stir in the taco seasoning and water.
3. Stir in the frozen cauliflower rice and can of diced tomatoes and chilies to the pan; simmer for about 10 minutes or until hot.
4. Top with cheddar cheese and allow it to melt.
5. Enjoy alone or with avocado, sour cream, jalapenos, lettuce or anything else you'd like.

Nutrition

Calories: 266 | Carbs: 11.7g |Protein: 29.5g | Fat: 11g | Sodium: 540mg |Fiber: 0.9g | Sugar: 6.7g

22. Easy Keto Pizza Chaffles

Prep Time: 15 minutes | Cook Time: 5 minutes | Serves : 2 mini pizzas

1 egg
14g ground almonds
100g shredded mozzarella
14g grated parmesan
1g Italian seasoning
0.5g garlic powder
pizza toppings of your choice

Instructions

1. Preheat your oven to 400 degrees and turn on your mini waffle maker.
2. In a small bowl, whisk the egg together and then combine with the rest of the ingredients.
3. Once your mini waffle maker is hot, sprinkle the griddle with a little shredded mozzarella.
4. Pour half of the batter in and then sprinkle with more cheese. Close the lid and cook until the automatic timer or light goes off; repeat for the next waffle.
5. Place the chaffles on a baking sheet and allow them to cool for a few minutes (so that they don't get soggy), and then spread with a low carb pizza sauce, shredded cheese and the toppings of your choice.
6. Bake for 3-4 minutes and then an additional minute or two with the broiler on to brown the cheese.
7. Sprinkle it with a little more Italian seasoning and enjoy!

Nutrition

Calories: 159 | Carbs: 3.8g| Protein: 9.5g |Fat: 11.6g | Sodium: 144mg | Fiber: 1.5g | Sugar: 0.2g

23. One Pot Low Carb and Keto Zuppa Toscana

Prep Time:5 minutes | Cook Time: 20minutes | Serves 8

1 diced small onion
450g mild Italian sausage
450g chopped kale
950g cauliflower fresh or frozen
6 chopped slices bacon
200g double cream

3 cloves garlic minced

950ml low sodium chicken stock

7g crushed red peppers optional

Salt and pepper to taste

Instructions
1. In a large pot over medium-high heat, brown sausage, and bacon. Once the meat is no longer pink, add the onion and garlic and saute for a few minutes.
2. Drain the excess fat and add in the cauliflower, chicken stock, crushed red pepper flakes and simmer on medium heat for 15 minutes or until the cauliflower is tender.
3. Reduce the heat and stir in the cream. Add the fresh kale or baby spinach, stir, and remove from heat.
4. Serve hot in big bowls topped with parmesan or extra crispy bacon bits and store the leftovers (in any) for up to 4 days.

Nutrition
Calories: 431 | Carbs: 5g | Protein: 13g |Fat: 40g |Sodium: 626mg |Fiber: 1g | Sugar: 2g

24.Thai Peanut Salad

Prep Time: 10 minutes | Total Time: 10 minutes | Serves 8

Salad
- 96g cabbage
- 64g cucumber
- 64g spring onions
- 71g salted peanuts
- 64g red bell pepper
- 340g diced cooked chicken

Thai Peanut Salad Dressing
- 89g peanut butter
- 44ml olive oil
- 44ml rice vinegar or regular vinegar
- 10g coconut aminos
- 4g granulated sugar substitute
- 6g garlic
- 1g ginger paste
- 3g red pepper flakes
- Salt and pepper to taste
- Optional: garnish with coriander

Instructions
1. In a large bowl add cabbage, cucumber, spring onions, peanuts, pepper, and chicken.
2. In a small bowl mix remaining ingredients.
3. Pour dressing over the salad and toss. Add salt and pepper to taste. 4. Enjoy!

Nutrition
Calories: 201| Carbs: 12g |Protein: 6.1g |Fat: 16.2| Sodium: 174.3mg|Fiber: 0.5g| Sugar: 3g

25. Minced Beef & Broccoli Casserole

Prep Time: 15 minutes | Cook Time: 40 minutes | Serves 4

- 450g extra lean minced beef
- 400g can tomato sauce
- 1400g small broccoli florets
- 400g cheddar cheese
- 6g finely grated parmesan cheese
- 1 chopped large stalk celery finely
- 9g table salt
- 3g garlic powder
- 2g ground cayenne

Instructions
1. Prepare: Preheat oven to 375 F. Cut any broccoli florets larger than 2 inches into smaller pieces, and add all broccoli to a large microwave-safe bowl. Cover and microwave until tender, about 5 minutes. Let them drain and steam out on paper towels.
2. Make Beef-Tomato Mixture: If wet, pat minced beef dry with paper towels. Add beef to a large pan over medium heat. Crumble beef with a stiff utensil, cook until browned, about 5 minutes. Keeping everything in the pan, stir in tomato sauce, celery, salt, garlic powder, and cayenne. Simmer for at least 10 minutes to thicken sauce, stirring occasionally. Turn off heat and let moisture steam out.
3. Assemble Casserole: Directly in an 8x8 inch baking dish, add broccoli, beef-tomato mixture, and half of cheddar cheese, carefully stirring together until well-mixed. Evenly top with remaining cheddar cheese. Sprinkle parmesan cheese on top.
4. Bake & Cool: Bake uncovered at 375 F until the casserole begins bubbling up sides and starts to brown on top, about 20 minutes. Let rest for about 10 minutes before cutting into it. Serve.

Nutrition
Calories: 370| Carbs: 9.5g| Protein: 37g|Fat: 19g|Sodium: 1290mg|Fiber: 4g|Sugar: 5.5g

26. Low Carb Steak Taco Bowl

Prep Time: 10 minutes | Cook Time: 15 minutes | Serves 2

7ml olive oil divided
3g minced garlic
¼ small onion sliced thinly or 5 - 6 spring onions
4 small portobello mushrooms sliced
½ small poblano pepper may use bell pepper
salt and pepper to taste
140g steak
4g taco seasoning mix
3g nacho cheese

Instructions

1. Heat 1-2 teaspoons of olive oil in a medium skillet and add garlic, onions, mushrooms and peppers. Cook until tender, about 10 minutes. Sprinkle it with salt and pepper, as desired. Remove from the skillet.
2. Add taco mix to sliced steak. Add 1 teaspoon olive oil to the skillet and heat over medium. Add steak and stir fry until brown and cooked- about 1-2 minutes depending on thickness of slices.
3. Add cooked veggies back to the skillet with steak and stir.
4. Heat queso and pour over the steak mixture.

Nutrition

Calories: 167 | Carbs: 3g | Protein: 18g | Fat: 9g | Sodium: 150mg | Fiber: 1g | Sugar: 2g

27. Pineapple Teriyaki Meatballs

Prep Time: 15 mins | Cook Time: 20 mins | Serves 4

570g minced turkey, 93% Lean
⅔ panko bread crumbs
1 large egg
1 small onion
1 clove garlic
2g coarse sea salt
0.5g freshly ground black pepper
Sauce
230g diced pineapple
108g soy sauce

233ml water
8g corn starch
2 cloves garlic
4g fresh ginger
1g red pepper flakes
optional garnish: green onion and sesame seeds

Instructions
1. Place all meatballs ingredients, except for onion and garlic, in a medium-sized bowl.
2. In a food processor or immersion blender cup, chop onion and garlic until fine. If you don't have this equipment, chop very finely with a knife. Add to the meatball mixture.
3. Mix until just combined (don't overmix--the meatball will be tough). Form into 24 balls, about one heaping tablespoon each. You could use a cookie scoop and place them on a cookie sheet, or use a mini muffin tin sprayed generously with cooking spray to portion them out.
4. Broil meatballs for 10 minutes.
5. While meatballs cook, add all teriyaki sauce ingredients to the same food processor or immersion blender cup. Blend until smooth.

Nutrition
Calories: 248 |Carbs: 16.6g | Protein 36.7g |Fat: 4.4g | Sodium: 620mg | Fiber: 1.6g | Sugar: 6.8g

28.Vegetable Hash with Spicy Salmon Bites

Prep Time: 20 minutes | Cook Time: 25 minutes | Serves 2

Vegetable hash
  15ml olive oil
  170g-230g brussel sprouts shaved
  1 onion slice
  220g broccoli florets
  220g asparagus cut into 3-cm pieces
  2 cloves garlic chopped small
  3g salt
  1g black pepper
  1 lemon cut into wedges
  15ml olive oil
  170g-230g salmon
  5g oregano

3g onion powder
2g garlic powder
2g salt
1g black pepper
3g paprika
3g cayenne pepper
6g kewpie mayonnaise or regular
14ml soy sauce
14ml sriracha
12g maple syrup

Instructions

1. Combine kewpie mayonnaise, sriracha, soy sauce and maple syrup in a small mixing bowl. Set aside.
2. Heat a 9-inch cast iron skillet or a non-stick skillet and add one tablespoon of olive oil.
3. Once the oil is hot, add the sliced onion and cut asparagus. Sauté for 1 minute.
4. Next, add the broccoli florets, chopped garlic, and shaved Brussel sprouts. Season with salt and black pepper.
5. Sauté until the vegetables have a light brown sear but are still slightly firm. Remove from heat.
6. Next, remove the pin bones from your salmon.
7. Option to remove the skin as well.
8. Cube the salmon and toss it with the blackening spice. Garlic powder, onion powder, dried oregano, cayenne pepper, black pepper, salt, and paprika.
9. Heat a second non-stick pan with olive oil over medium heat.
10. Once well coated, add the seasoned salmon bites to the second pan.
11. Sear until golden brown.

Nutrition

Calories: 577 |Carbs: 32g |Protein: 26g |Fat: 41g |Sodium: 1805mg| Fiber:9g| Sugar:13g

29. Coriander Lime Grilled Prawns

Prep Time: 30 minutes | Cook Time: 5 minutes | Serves 3

230g prawns
30g lime juice
1/2 fruit (5cm dia) Limes
8ml olive oil
1g fresh coriander
1/4 pepper Jalapeno peppers

1/2 cloves, minced Garlic
1g dash salt
0.5g dash pepper

Instructions
1. Marinate the prawns in the mixture of the lime juice, zest, oil, coriander, jalapeno, garlic, salt, and pepper for 30 minutes to overnight.
2. Skewer the prawns and grill over medium-high heat until cooked, about 2-3 minutes per side.

Nutrition
Calories: 121 | Carbs: 4.4g | Fat: 4.6g | Protein: 15.7g | Sodium: 160mg | Fiber: 0.6g | Sugar: 1g

30. Lemon Prawns with Garlic Olive Oil

Prep time: 5 minutes | Cook time: 6 minutes | Serves 4

454g medium prawns, cleaned and deveined
92ml olive oil, divided
Juice of ½ lemon
3 garlic cloves, minced and divided
3g salt
1g red pepper flakes
Lemon wedges, for serving (optional)
Ready-made tomato sauce, for dipping (optional)

Instructions
1. Preheat the air fryer to 380°F(193°C).
2. In a large bowl, combine the shrimp with 30ml the olive oil, as well as the lemon juice, ⅓ of the minced garlic, salt, and red pepper flakes. Toss to coat the shrimp well.
3. In a small ramekin, combine the remaining 62ml olive oil and the remaining minced garlic.
4. Tear off a 12-by-12-inch sheet of aluminum foil. Pour the shrimp into the center of the foil, then fold the sides up and crimp the edges so that it forms an aluminum foil bowl that is open on top. Place this packet into the air fryer basket.
5. Roast the shrimp for 4 minutes, then open the air fryer and place the ramekin with oil and garlic in the basket beside the shrimp packet. Cook for 2 more minutes.

6. Transfer the shrimp on a serving plate or platter with the ramekin of garlic olive oil on the side for dipping. You may also serve with lemon wedges and marinara sauce, if desired.

Per Serving

Calories: 283| carbs: 1g| protein: 23g | fat: 21g | sodium: 427mg| fiber: 0g | Sugar:1g

CHAPTER 3   DINNER

1. Fluffy Omelet with Cheese and Courgette

Prep Time: 10 minutes | Cook Time: 5 minutes | Serves 3

28g butter
3 extra large Egg
21g cheddar cheese
2g salt
1g pepper
1/2 small courgette

Instructions

1. Preheat the broiler to high temperature.
2. Heat a 10 inch (25cm) nonstick frying pan over medium heat and add butter. Once the butter sizzles, pour in egg mixture evenly over the pan. Reduce heat to low and cook until set and golden brown (about 5 minutes).
3. Remove the pan from heat and sprinkle the top of the omelet with cheese, shredded courgette, salt, and pepper. Place the omelet in a frying pan under the broiler and cook until the cheese melts, about 1-2 mins.
4. Remove the frying pan from the broiler. Gently fold the omelet in half and serve.

Nutrition

Calories: 540 | Carbs: 3.4g | Fat: 46.4g | Protein: 27.2g | Sodium: 84mg | Fiber: 0.6g | Sugar: 8g

2. Artichoke Chicken

Prep Time: 10 minutes | Cook Time: 30 minutes | Serves 6

6 boneless skinless chicken breast halves

1 can water-packed artichoke hearts
150g grated parmesan cheese
174g mayonnaise
2 garlic cloves minced

Instructions

1. Preheat oven to 375 degrees and spray a 13x9 inch baking dish with cooking spray. Salt and pepper the chicken breast halves and place in the dish.
2. In a bowl, combine the artichoke hearts, parmesan cheese, mayonnaise and garlic.
3. Stir together until combined.
4. Spread artichoke mixture over chicken breasts.
5. Bake, uncovered, 30-35 minutes or until chicken juices run clear and top starts to slightly brown.

Nutrition

Calories: 481 | Fat: 29.8g | Carbs: 3.5g | Sodium:1828mg | Protein: 44.3g | Sugar:5g

3. Low Carb Hamburger Stroganoff

Prep Time: 15 minutes | Cook Time: 15 minutes | Serves 2

7g butter
1/2 cloves, minced Garlic
110g minced beef
0.5g salt
0.3g pepper
56g mushrooms
19g water
72g sour cream
13g paprika
5ml lemon juice

Instructions

1. Melt 14g butter in a pan then add garlic and salute until garlic is golden.
2. Add the beef, season with salt and pepper, then cook until browned. Remove beef from pan and set aside.
3. Melt another tablespoon of butter in the pan. Add mushrooms and wine/water and cook until liquid is reduced by about half and mushrooms are softened.
4. Remove pan from heat and mix in sour cream and paprika. Return the pan to low heat. Stir in lemon juice and meat. Add more seasoning if needed.

Nutrition

Calories: 328 | Carbs: 3.1g| Protein: 15.2g | Fat: 28.5g | Sodium: 102mg | Fiber: 0.4g | Sugar: 1.8g

4. Quick Italian Eggs

Prep Time: 5minutes | Cook Time: 5minutes | Serves 1

2 eggs
64g ready-made tomato sauce
15g spinach(roughly chopped)
32g mozzarella cheese
Salt and pepper to taste

Instructions

1. Pour ready-made tomato sauce to a small sauté pan.
2. Add the spinach and break in the eggs.
3. Season with salt and pepper.
4. Top with cheese.
5. Put the pan on the stove at medium to high heat.
6. As soon as the Marinara starts bubbling, cover and cook for 3 - 5 minutes.
7. We cooked ours for 4 minutes and it gave a medium egg.

Nutrition

Calories: 121 | Carbs: 4g |Protein: 10g | Fat: 7g | Sodium: 477mg | Fiber: 1g | Sugar: 3g

5. Steak Kebabs with Chimichurri

Prep Time: 15 minutes | Cook Time: 10 minutes | Serves 6

567g beef
fresh ground pepper
6g coarse sea salt
1 large red onion cut into large chunks
18 cherry tomatoes
6 bamboo skewers soaked in water for 1 hour

For the Chimichurri Sauce:
- 2 chopped packed tbsp parsley finely
- 2 packed tbsp chopped coriander
- 28g red onion
- 1 clove garlic minced
- 30ml extra virgin olive oil
- 30ml apple cider vinegar
- 15ml water
- 1g coarse sea salt
- 6g fresh black pepper
- 0.5g crushed red pepper flakes

Instructions

1. Season the meat with salt and pepper.
2. For the chimichurri, combine the red onion, vinegar, salt and olive oil and let it sit for about 5 minutes. Add the remaining ingredients and mix; set aside in the refrigerator until ready to use.
3. Place the onions, beef and tomatoes onto the skewers.
4. Prepare the grill on high heat. Grill the steaks to desired doneness, about 2 to 3 minutes per side for medium-rare. Transfer steaks to a platter and top with chimichurri sauce.

Nutrition

Calories: 219 | Carbs: 5.5g | Protein: 20g | Fat: 13g | Sodium: 335.5mg | Fiber: 1g

6. Garlic Butter Pork Chops with Courgette

Prep Time: 10 minutes | Cook Time: 25 minutes | Serves 4

For the Pork Chops & Courgette
- 4 pork chops 1-cm thick
- salt and fresh ground pepper, to taste
- 2g paprika
- 28g butter
- 22ml vegetable oil
- 2 courgette sliced into half moons
- 56g butter
- 5g garlic powder
- 5g dried basil
- 2g dried parsley
- 4g dried oregano

Instructions

1. Season pork chops with salt, pepper, and paprika. Cut a few slits in the fat surrounding the pork chops. This will help with keeping the chops from curling up while frying.
2. Heat butter and 1 tablespoon vegetable oil in a large skillet set over medium-high heat. Add the pork chops to the hot oil and cook for 5 minutes per side, or until cooked through. Pork chops are cooked through when internal temperature reaches 140°F. Use an instant read thermometer for best results.
3. Also, cooking time will depend on the thickness of the pork chops; they should be up to 1/2-inch thick.
4. Prepare the garlic butter by combining butter, garlic powder, dried basil, dried parsley, and dried oregano; mash with a fork until thoroughly incorporated.
5. Remove pork chops from skillet; keep covered.
6. Set the skillet over medium-high heat and add remaining oil. Add courgette slices to the hot oil; season with salt and pepper, and cook for 2 to 3 minutes, or until tender. Remove from the skillet.
7. Transfer pork chops and courgette to a serving plate. Add a dollop of garlic butter to each pork chop and serve!

Nutrition

Calories: 508 | Carbs: 5g | Protein: 37g | Fat: 38g | Sodium: 253mg | Fiber: 2g | Sugar: 3g

7. Pesto Salmon

Prep Time: 5 minutes | Cook Time: 15 minutes | Serves 4

660g multicolored cherry tomatoes
1 medium shallot thinly sliced
30ml extra-virgin olive oil
2g salt
4 skin-on salmon fillets
85g refrigerated basil pesto
32g shaved parmesan cheese
18g pine nuts
28g chopped fresh basil

Instructions

1. Preheat oven to 425°F. Coat a large rimmed baking sheet with cooking spray. Combine tomatoes, shallot, oil and salt in a large bowl; stir until well coated.

2. Place salmon fillets, skin-side down, on the prepared baking sheet. Spread 1 1/2 tablespoons pesto on top of each fillet. Scatter the tomato mixture evenly around the salmon.
3. Bake until the tomatoes have started to soften and burst and the salmon is just cooked through, 12 to 14 minutes. Arrange the salmon and the tomato mixture on 4 plates. Top evenly with Parmesan, pine nuts and basil.

Nutrition

Calories: 446| Carbs: 11g | Protein: 34g | fat: 30g |sodium: 412mg | fiber: 3g | sugar: 7g

8. Chipotle Air Fryer Chicken Thighs

Prep Time: 10 minutes | Cook Time: 25 minutes | Serves 2

4 bone-in skin-on chicken thighs
14g baking powder
2g garlic powder
1g-2g fine sea salt
1g smoked paprika
1g chipotle powder
4g coconut oil

Instructions

1. Preheat your air fryer to 360°F (make sure to remove the air fryer rack before preheating). Place the chicken pieces on a plate lined with paper towels and pat them dry completely. Place the dry chicken on a clean, dry plate.
2. In a small dish, mix the baking powder and seasonings. Generously sprinkle the chicken with the seasoning mix, turning it over to season both sides. Gently pat it or spread it around so it's even.
3. Rub a bit of oil onto the removable air fryer rack to prevent the chicken from sticking. Place the chicken thighs on the rack, skin side down. Air fry for 15 minutes at 360° (if the thighs are extra large, go for 20 minutes), then remove the air fryer basket.
4. Flip the chicken so it is now skin side up and place the basket back inside the air fryer. Turn the temperature up to 390°F and air fry for another 5-10 minutes, or until the skin is golden brown and the chicken is done (check it after 5 minutes). It will have an internal temp of at least 165°F. If the chicken needs to cook longer, add increments of 4 minutes at a time. The air fry time will vary based on the size of your chicken thighs. If they're extra large, the initial cook time will likely be 20 minutes (at 360°F).

Nutrition

Calories: 146 |Carbs: 2g | Protein: 8g|Fat: 13g | Sodium: 971mg| Fiber: 0g | Sugar: 0g

9. Low Carb Aubergine Pizza

Prep Time: 10 minutes | Cook Time 15 minutes | Serves 4

1 large aubergine
15ml olive oil
236ml no sugar added pizza sauce
2 garlic cloves minced
½ yellow onion sliced
96g fresh baby spinach sea salt
177ml shredded mozzarella cheese
38g chopped fresh oregano crushed red pepper

Instructions
1. Preheat: Preheat the oven to 400°F.
2. Cut aubergine: Slice the aubergine lengthwise, about 1/4-1/3 inch thick. Brush or rub a little olive oil on each side of the aubergine slices and place on a baking sheet lined with parchment paper. Sprinkle it with salt and pepper. Place in the oven for 7-10 minutes, or until aubergine is hot and starting to cook down.
3. Meanwhile grab a skillet, add 7 ml olive oil and sauté the garlic and onion until soft (about 3-4 minutes). Season with salt and pepper. Add pizza sauce and spinach to the skillet and cook for 1-2 additional minutes until mixture is warm and spinach has wilted.
4. Remove the aubergine slices from the oven, top each with the onion and spinach mixture. Sprinkle it with cheese and chopped oregano. Place in the oven for approximately 5 minutes, or until the cheese has melted.
5. Serve immediately with more fresh oregano and crushed red pepper.

Nutrition
Calories: 331| Carbs: 25g| Protein: 17g |Fat: 19g | Sodium: 791mg | Fiber: 9g|Sugar: 15g

10. Mexican Taco Stuffed Courgette Boats

Prep Time 20 minutes | Cook Time 40 minutes| Servings 8 boats

4 courgette squash about the same size
45ml olive oil
1.4g salt
1 chopped bell pepper finely
1 chopped sweet onion finely

2 cloves garlic crushed

454g minced meat beef

1g homemade taco seasoning

1.4g pepper

59ml salsa mild or medium

236ml shredded cheese divided

Instructions

1. Preheat the oven to 400 degrees.
2. Cut both the stem and the blossom ends off of each courgette and slice in half lengthwise. Scoop the seeds out using a spoon with a slightly sharp edge, leaving about ½-inch of courgette around all sides. (Reserve the courgette flesh that was scooped out.)
3. Drizzle 15 ml of oil over all of the insides of the courgette boats and sprinkle with 1.42 g of salt. Place courgette flat-side down on a large baking sheet in a single layer and bake in a preheated oven for 10 minutes.
4. Saute chopped bell pepper, onion, salt, and pepper in 28.3g of oil over medium heat in a large stainless steel skillet for 2-3 minutes.
5. Add 1 cup of chopped courgette flesh that was previously removed from the boats, and 2 cloves of crushed garlic. Continue sauteeing for an additional 1-2 minutes.
6. Push vegetables to the side of the skillet and add minced meat. Cook for 7-10 minute or until meat is completely cooked through. Drain any excess liquid from the pan when the meat is done cooking.
7. Turn off heat and mix in seasoning ingredients, salsa, and shredded cheese. . Flip over all of the pre-baked courgette boats so the hollow cavity is facing up and fill all 8 courgette boats with equal amounts of the minced meat taco filling mixture. Sprinkle it with the remaining cheese.
8. Return the courgette to the oven and cook for an additional 10-15 minutes. . Serve with chopped spring onions or coriander and enjoy

Nutrition

Calories: 553 | Carbs:59.6g|Protein 35.1g | Fat: 20.3g| Sodium: 3713 m |Sugar: 3.3g

11. Crustless Cheesy Chicken and Asparagus Pie

Prep Time:15 minutes | Cook Time 45 minutes | Serves 4

250g cooked chicken

2 white onions [chopped]

400g can asparagus

125g cheddar cheese

2g paprika
1g mustard powder
2g garlic powder
6g salt [we used regular fine table salt]
1g white pepper pinch cayenne pepper
118ml milk
4 large eggs
15ml oil [of choice for cooking and greasing your pie dish

Instructions

1. Preheat the oven to 350F/180C
2. Cook the onion in a little bit of oil until it starts to brown, 10-15 minutes. Use the time while the onion cooks to prepare the rest of the ingredients, but remember to stir the onions every minute or so.
3. Once the onions are nicely browned, add the chicken and all the spices into the pan and stir until everything is well combined
4. Use a paper towel to wipe a bit of oil on the inside of your pie dish.
5. Now, add the onion and chicken to the pie dish.
6. Add the asparagus pieces on top and gently mix. .
7. Top with the shredded cheese.
8. Now, in a small bowl, mix together the milk and eggs and carefully pour over the ingredients in the pie dish. Be sure to gently shake the dish a little bit to help the egg mix spread into all the nooks and crannies.
9. Slide into the oven and bake for 45 minutes.
10. When done, allow to stand for 5-10 minutes before serving

Nutrition

Calories: 318 | Carbs: 8g | Protein: 26g | Fat: 20g | Sodium: 901mg| Fiber: 1g | Sugar: 4g

12. Salmon in Roasted Pepper Sauce

Prep Time: 5 minutes | Cook Time: 20 minutes | Serves 2

2 salmon fillets skin on
Salt and pepper to taste
15ml olive oil
14g butter
3 diced cloves garlic finely
113g diced roasted red peppers
120g fresh baby spinach
119g double cream

32g grated Parmesan cheese
1.2ml red pepper flakes or to taste
15g chopped parsley
Salt and pepper to taste

Instructions

1. Season the salmon fillets with salt and pepper.
2. Heat the oil in a medium non-stick skillet over medium heat. Cook the salmon fillets flesh side down first, for 5 minutes on each side, or until cooked to your liking. Once cooked, remove them from the pan and set aside.
3. To the same pan, add butter and garlic. Cook for 1 minute, add the roasted peppers, and cook for 2 more minutes.
4. Add the spinach and allow it to wilt.
5. Reduce the heat to low, and add Half & Half, Parmesan, red pepper flakes, parsley, salt, and pepper. Stir and bring to a simmer. .
6. Return the salmon to the pan and spoon the sauce over each filet.
7. Serve over pasta, rice, or steamed vegetables.

Nutrition

Calories: 527 | Carbs:10g | Protein: 43g| Fat: 35g| Sodium: 2345mg |Fiber:2g | Sugar: 1g

13.Chicken Fried Cauliflower Rice

Prep Time:15 minutes | Cook Time: 15 minutes | Serves 2

- 1 small head of cauliflower
- 2 cubed chicken breasts
- 1 diced onion
- 250g frozen mixed vegetables
- 2 eggs beaten
- 4g sesame oil to taste
- 4g soy sauce

Instructions

1. In a pan, cook the egg, seasoned with a little bit of soy sauce. Remove and set aside.
2. In the same pan, sauté the onion until soft in a little bit of oil. Use a high heat.
3. Add the chicken and garlic and sauté until the chicken is almost cooked, about 3-5 minutes.
4. Add the grated cauliflower, frozen mixed vegetables, soy sauce and sesame oil.
5. Cook until the cauliflower and vegetables soften, another 5 - 10 minutes.
6. At the very end, add the egg back into the skillet and stir until evenly spread.

7. Garnish with chopped spring onions and serve immediately with homemade white sauce.

Nutrition
Calories: 245 | Carbs: 16g | Protein: 31.3g | Fat: 6.69g| Fiber: 5.16g | Sugar: 4g

14. Orange Chicken Salad

Prep Time:15 minutes | Cook Time: 10 minutes | Serves 4

- 454g chicken breast
- 120g lettuce
- 165g cherry tomatoes
- 2 avocado
- 64g raw pecan nuts
- 1 garlic clove
- 4g dried thyme
- 2 oranges
- 75g butter
- 15ml oil

Instructions
1. Divide the lettuce into plates and add cherry tomatoes and avocado on top. Set aside.
2. In a sauté pan, over a high heat: Add the chicken strips, garlic, thyme, salt and pepper, and cook until the chicken is seared and cooked through, approximately 5 minutes.
3. Squeeze the juice of the oranges over the chicken and as soon as it boils vigorously, remove the pan from the heat and stir the cold butter into the sauce. This will thicken it.
4. Now, add the chicken to the salad and top with the pecan nuts.
5. Lastly, pour the pan sauce over the salad or keep on the side.
6. Serve immediately.

Nutrition
Calories: 592 |Carbs: 22g |Protein: 29g |Fat: 46g |Sodium: 285mg|Fiber: 11g|Sugar:10g

15. Cuban Mojo Chicken

Prep Time: 15 minutes | Cook Time: 35 minutes | Serves 4

- 4 bone-in chicken leg quarters
- 118ml orange juice
- ⅓ lime juice
- 3 garlic cloves

32g coriander
1 lime zest
3g cumin
6g dried oregano
6g salt
3g black ground pepper
118ml olive oil
1 onion quartered
½ avocado
113g diced pineapple
82g cherry tomatoes
64g black beans rinsed and drained
250g steamed rice

Instructions

1. Preheat oven at 350°F
2. Add to the food processor, orange juice, lime juice, garlic, coriander, lime zest, cumin, oregano, salt, and black ground pepper. 118 ml orange juice, ⅓ lime juice, 3 garlic cloves, 32g coriander, 1 lime zest, 14g cumin, 6g dried oregano, 6g salt, 3g black ground pepper
3. Process for 10 seconds. You don't want the sauce to become too creamy.
4. Add the olive oil and process for 5 seconds, just to combine ever so slightly. ½ cup olive oil
5. Add the chicken and chopped onion in a large bowl.
6. Pour half of the mojo sauce over the chicken and onions. Cover with cling film, and marinate in the fridge for 3 hours.
7. Set aside the remaining half of the mojo sauce for later use.
8. When the chicken is done marinating, add chicken and onions to the baking tray, together with the sauce it marinated in.
9. Bake at 350°F for 35-40 minutes.

Pineapple-Avocado Salsa

1. Meanwhile, chop up the pineapple, avocado, and cherry tomatoes into small pieces and add them in a small bowl. Mix in the remaining half of Mojo sauce you saved earlier. Your salsa is ready! ½ avocado, 112g pineapple, 63g cherry tomatoes
2. Drizzle pineapple-avocado salsa over baked chicken, serve with steamed rice and beans, and enjoy!

Nutrition

Calories: 674 |Carbs: 32g |Protein: 28g |Fat: 55g|Sodium: 784mg|Fiber: 5g |Sugar: 7g

16. Coriander Lime Chicken

Prep Time: 25 minute | Cook Time: 10 minutes | Marinate: 2 hours | Serves 6

- 680g boneless skinless chicken breasts
- 177ml freshly squeezed orange juice
- 118ml olive oil
- 78ml freshly squeezed lime juice
- 3g lime zest
- 21g honey
- 6g cumin
- 37ml soy sauce
- 8.4g minced garlic
- 43g coarsely chopped coriander
- 1 ripe mango
- 1 ripe avocado
- 32g finely diced red onion
- 32g finely chopped red pepper
- 14g finely chopped jalapeno

Instructions

1. Marinade: Whisk together all of the marinade ingredients in a medium-sized bowl: orange juice, olive oil, lime juice, lime zest, honey, cumin, soy sauce, garlic, and coriander. Add salt and pepper to taste. Reserve about 118 ml of marinade, and pour the rest into a large resealable bag.
2. Trim the chicken fat. Pound the breasts to even thickness or slice in half to get evenly sized breasts and place in the bag with the rest of the marinade. Refrigerate for at least 30 minutes, making sure to flip the bag halfway through. I recommend marinating for 2-8 hours.
3. Lightly oil the grill grate or grill ridges on a grill pan or add 14g of oil to a skillet and then place the marinated chicken on the grill. Discard leftover marinade.
4. Grill for 10-12 minutes or until chicken juices run clear and internal temperature is at 165 degrees F. Flip the chicken halfway and brush it generously with the reserved 118 ml marinade.
5. Mango Salsa : Take 14g orange juice, 5ml olive oil, 14ml lime juice, lime zest, and 32g coriander and toss together.
6. Chop the mango and avocado into bite-sized pieces. Add to the salsa along with the finely chopped red onion, red pepper, and jalapeño. Season the salsa to taste with pepper, salt, and remaining 6g cumin and stir to mix.
7. Assembly: Serve grilled chicken over a bed of coriander-lime rice or quinoa and add spoonfuls of the salsa on top. Enjoy immediately!

Nutrition

Calories: 430 | Carbs: 18g | Protein: 27g | Fat: 29g | Sodium: 557mg | Fiber: 3g | Sugar: 12g

17. Baked Coconut Lime Chicken

Prep Time: 10 minutes | Cook Time: 20 minutes | Serves 3

- 453g boneless skinless chicken breasts about 4 total chicken breasts
- 30g plain flour
- 32g chopped coriander
- 26g coconut oil
- 15ml olive oil
- 1 garlic clove minced
- 237ml coconut milk
- 157ml chicken stock
- 9g brown sugar or sub coconut sugar
- 2 limes
- 1 green onion chopped for garnish salt and pepper to taste

Instructions

1. Preheat the oven to 375°.
2. Heat a large, oven-safe skillet or dutch oven over medium heat, then add the coconut oil and olive oil.
3. Combine the flour and coriander in a bowl, then dip each chicken breast into the mixture until coated, placing it directly into the hot skillet. Pan-sear the chicken for 3-4 minutes per side, or until lightly browned. Once the chicken is almost done, add the minced garlic and let it cook down for 30 seconds or so.
4. While the chicken is searing, mix the coconut milk, stock, sugar, and juice from 1 lime in a bowl.
5. Remove skillet from the heat, then pour the coconut milk mixture over top of the chicken. Place the skillet into the oven and bake the chicken for 10-15 minutes, or until the chicken reaches an internal temperature of 165°.
6. Remove skillet from the oven, and drizzle the remaining lime juice (juice from 1 lime) over the chicken. Sprinkle everything with salt, pepper, extra chopped coriander and chopped onion.

Nutrition

Calories: 464 | Carbs: 14g | Protein: 51g | Fat: 28g | Sodium: 416mg | Fiber: 1g | Sugar: 4g

18. Keto Cheesy Burger Stuffed Portobellos

Prep Time: 10 minutes | Cook Time: 20 minutes | Serves 1

1 mushroom, whole Mushrooms
140g minced beef
56g cheddar cheese
15g spinach
5g parmesan cheese
2g salt
2g pepper

Instructions

1. Preheat the oven to 375F degrees.
2. Remove the stems from the portobellos. Chop stems finely and add to the minced beef. With a spoon, scrape out the gills on the underside of the mushrooms and discard.
3. Finely chop spinach and grate cheese. Set aside.
4. Season the mushrooms with a sprinkling of salt and pepper. Mix the cheddar cheese and spinach into the minced beef. Season with a dash of salt and pepper. Form two patties and press them onto the portobello mushrooms.
5. Place the stuffed mushrooms on a small sheet pan or baking dish and cook for 20 minutes or until cooked through. Add the Parmesan cheese to the top of each and pop back into the oven to melt the cheese or under the broiler to brown. Serve hot and enjoy

Nutrition

Calories: 744 | Carbs: 5.3g | Fat: 63.4g | Protein: 37.6g| Sodium:884mg | Fiber: 1.4g

19. Keto Chili

Prep Time: 5 minutes | Cook Time: 20 minutes | Serves 6

680g minced beef lean
1 chopped medium sized Yellow Onion
3 cloves garlic minced
9g avocado oil
1 medium sized Bell Pepper chopped
2 chopped small Jalapenos de-seeded and
3 diced medium sized plum tomatoes
29ml keto ketchup or tomato sauce
473ml beef stock low sodium
29.6g chili seasoning
1g cayenne pepper

3g ground cumin
1g ground cinnamon
1g smoked paprika
2g garlic powder
3g Onion powder
1g Ginger powder
2 dried bay leaves
6g salt

Instructions

1. Heat a Pan over medium high heat. Add Avocado Oil or any cooking oil in it. As the oil shimmers, add the Onion & Garlic. Cook for 2-3 min. Add the meat and cook until it browns for 3-4 min.
2. Add the remaining ingredients and the spices. Toss to combine. As the chili comes to a boil, cover with a lid. Reduce the heat to low. Let the Chili simmer over low heat for 10-15 min. Stir occasionally.
3. Once the Chili has thickened, serve in a bowl. Garnish with your desired toppings and serve

Nutrition

Calories:368 |Carbs: 8g |Protein: 23g |Fat: 27g |Sodium: 821mg |Fiber: 2g |Sugar: 3g

20. Low Carb Mushroom & Spinach Cauliflower Rice

Prep Time: 5 minutes | Cook Time: 20 minutes | Serves: 3

284g frozen riced cauliflower
14ml soy sauce
15ml olive oil
50g chopped onion
2 minced garlic cloves
709g sliced mushrooms
60g spinach

Instructions

1. Cook cauliflower rice according to instructions on the package.
2. Heat olive oil in a skillet and add onions and cook until soft.
3. Toss in mushrooms and saute until cooked.
4. Now add garlic, and stir.
5. Add cauliflower rice and soy sauce. Stir until cauliflower rice has absorbed soy sauce.
6. Top mixture with spinach, stir and cook until wilted.

Nutrition

Calories:100 |Fat: 4.1g | Carbs: 11.5g |Protein: 7.7g| Sodium: 294mg |Fiber: 3.7g| Sugar: 5g

21. Garlic Parmesan Brussels Sprouts with Bacon

Prep Time:10 minutes | Cook Time: 30 minutes | Serves 6

- 6 strips of bacon
- 680g brussels sprouts
- 3 cloves of garlic minced
- 238g double cream
- 64g shredded mozzarella cheese
- 32g grated parmesan cheese
- 3g salt
- 1.42g black pepper

Instructions

1. In a large pan over medium-high heat, cook bacon for about 5 minutes until crispy. Drain, chop and set aside.
2. To the same pan, in about 2 tbsp of reserved bacon fat, saute brussels sprouts for about 6- 8 minutes. Add the garlic, and saute for 1 minute more until the garlic is fragrant.
3. Add the double cream, and simmer for 4-6 minutes.
4. Add the cheeses and stir to melt. And salt and pepper to taste. Add back the bacon, and serve.

Nutrition

Calories: 273 | Carbs: 11g |Protein: 11g | Fat: 22g| Sodium:549mg| Fiber: 3g | Sugar: 3g

22. Crustless Taco Pie

Prep Time: 20 minutes | Cook Time: 40 minutes | Serves 4

- 454g minced beef
- 42.5g taco seasoning
- 159g double cream
- 4 large eggs
- 43g chunky salsa
- 32g cheddar cheese
- 3g garlic salt
- 0.5g ground black pepper

Instructions

1. Preheat an oven to 350F, making sure the oven rack is in the center position. Grease a 9" pie pan. Set the pan aside.
2. Brown the minced beef in a skillet, adding oil if needed to keep it from sticking, until it's cooked through. Drain any extra grease.
3. Add the taco seasoning to the minced beef in the same pan and stir it to combine. Spoon the taco beef into the greased pie pan.
4. In a small bowl, combine the double cream and eggs together, and then add the salsa, 1 cup of shredded cheese, garlic salt, and pepper.
5. Pour the egg mixture over the top of the taco beef in the pie pan. Top with an additional 1/4 cup of shredded cheese.
6. Bake the keto taco pie uncovered for 35 to 40 minutes, or until the center is set and the top is golden brown.
7. Let your crustless taco pie cool 5 minutes before serving.
8. Add optional garnishes, if desired, like sour cream, salsa, coriander, chives, avocado, diced tomatoes, or olives. Enjoy!

Nutrition

Calories: 329 | Carbs: 4g | Protein: 23g |Fat: 24g | Sodium: 591mg| Fiber: 1g|Sugar: 2g

23. Chipotle Honey Chicken Skewers

Prep Time: 10 minutes | Cook Time: 12 minutes | Makes: 8 skewers

- 907g boneless and skinless chicken breasts
- 170g honey raw preferred
- 28g tomato paste
- 59ml apple cider vinegar
- 6g chipotle chili powder
- 1 chopped garlic clove very finely
- 3g salt

Instructions

1. Slice chicken into very thin strips with a very sharp knife. Thread accordion-style onto wooden skewers.
2. In a small bowl, whisk together honey, tomato paste, apple cider vinegar, chipotle chili powder, chopped garlic, and optional salt. Spoon sauce over skewers.
3. Add skewers to a hot grill and cook for 10-12 minutes, or until chicken is fully cooked, basting with sauce and turning every 2-3 minutes to evenly cook the entire skewer of chicken.

4. Alternately, the skewers can be baked in an oven preheated to 400 degrees for 16-18 minutes, or until fully cooked.

Nutrition
Calories: 193| Carbs: 18.8g |Protein: 26.6g|Fat: 1.7g| Sodium: 235mg |Fiber: 0.5g | Sugar: 18g

24. Chicken Mushroom Soup
Prep Time: 10 minutes | Cook Time: 35 minutes | Serves 7

- 30ml olive oil
- 1134g chicken breast cut into 1-inch pieces
- 6g salt and pepper
- 454g Button mushrooms
- 227g Baby portobello mushrooms
- 227g shiitake mushrooms
- 1 chopped large yellow onion
- 6 garlic cloves minced
- 1 package thyme leaves left on the stem rinsed dried and tied into
- 10 chopped sage leaves rinsed dried and finely
- 74ml sweet Marsala wine
- 1182ml chicken stock
- 170g cream cheese
- 64g grated Parmesan cheese
- 43g shredded Monterey Jack cheese
- 2-3 bundles with kitchen twine

Instructions
1. Add olive oil to a Dutch oven or large pot over medium high heat. Add the chicken and cook for 10 minutes, then remove the chicken from the pan with a slotted spoon and set aside.
2. Add all the mushrooms and saute for 6 minutes. Reserve 28g of cooked mushrooms for garnish if you desire.
3. Add onions, garlic, thyme, sage, Marsala wine, and saute 4 more minutes.
4. Next, add the chicken stock and bring to a simmer. Then stir in the chicken and simmer for 10 minutes uncovered.
5. Remove the thyme stems from the pot and discard. Whisk in the cream cheese, Parmesan cheese and Monterey jack cheese until smooth.
6. You can pan fry the reserved mushrooms in a little olive oil to use for garnish.
7. Garnish with extra mushrooms, sour cream, Monterey jack cheese, and parsley

Nutrition
Calories: 476 | Carbs:12g |Protein: 48g |Fat: 23g|Sodium: 660mg | Fiber: 2g | Sugar: 8g

25. Spinach and Ricotta Hasselback Chicken

Prep Time: 10 minutes | Cook Time: 25 minutes | Serves 1 ½

- 3ml Olive oil
- 340g Chicken breast
- 45g Spinach
- 45g Ricotta cheese
- 3g Salt
- 2g Pepper
- 21g Cheddar cheese
- 2g Paprika

Instructions

1. Preheat the oven to 400 degrees F.
2. Heat oil in a skillet over medium heat. Wilt spinach, 2-3 minutes; add ricotta and cook for 30-60 seconds and mix.
3. Slice chicken halfway through in several places across the top of the breast, season with salt and pepper, and stuff with the spinach/ricotta mixture.
4. Add shredded cheese on top, and sprinkle with paprika.
5. Bake for 20-25 minutes or until chicken is cooked through and no longer pink.
6. Serve immediately and enjoy!

Nutrition
Calories:412 | Carbs: 2.8g| Fat: 17.1g |Protein: 58.8g | Sodium:1868mg | Fiber:1g

26. Caprese Chicken

Prep time: 10 minutes | Cook Time: 15 minutes | Serves 4

- 4 (170g) chicken breasts
- 8g italian seasoning
- 10g sea or coarse sea salt
- 3g garlic powder
- 6g onion powder
- 6g cracked black pepper
- 15ml olive oil
- 227g fresh mozzarella sliced into 8 even pieces

2 vine ripened tomatoes sliced into ½" slices

fresh basil - taste aged balsamic or balsamic glaze to taste

Instructions

1. Prepare the chicken. Place one chicken breast onto a sheet of parchment paper. Fold the paper over the chicken. Using a rolling pin, pound the chicken breast to even thickness of a little less than 1". Set aside and repeat with the remaining chicken breasts.
2. Combine the italian seasoning, sea salt, garlic powder, onion powder, and pepper in a small bowl. Stir to combine.
3. Brush the chicken with olive oil, then sprinkle with the seasoning blend. Flip the chicken oven, then oil and season the other side.
4. Heat a grill or grill pan over high heat. Place the chicken breasts onto the grill and cook 5- 6 minutes per side, or until the internal temperature reads 155°F using an instant read thermometer (the chicken will come to proper temperature in the next step).
5. Top each chicken breast with 2 slices fresh mozzarella. Continue grilling 3 minutes, or until the cheese is melted and the internal temperature reads 165°F.
6. Place the chicken breasts onto a platter or individual plates. Top each chicken breast with 2-3 slices of fresh tomatoes, then sprinkle with fresh basil and additional salt and pepper to taste. Just before serving, drizzle with aged balsamic vinegar or balsamic reduction. Serve immediately

Nutrition

Calories: 391 | Carbs: 8g | Protein: 49g | Fat: 18g | Sodium: 1169mg|Fiber: 2g| Sugar: 3g

27 Fried Steak and Asparagus Bundles

Prep Time: 15 minutes | Cook Time: 15 minutes | Serves 6

907–1134g Flank steak

Coarse sea salt and black pepper, to taste

118ml Tamari sauce

2 cloves garlic - crushed

454g asparagus

3 bell peppers - seeded and sliced thinly

59ml balsamic vinegar

78ml beef stock

28g unsalted butter

Olive oil spray

Instructions

1. Season steaks with salt and pepper.
2. Place steaks into a large zip top bag. Add: Tamari sauce and garlic. Seal bag.

3. Massage steaks so that they're completely coated. Transfer to refrigerator and allow to marinade for a minimum of 1 hour up to overnight.
4. When ready to assemble, remove steaks from marinade and place on a cutting board or sheet. Discard marinade.
5. Equally divide and then place asparagus and bell peppers into the middle of each piece of steak.
6. Roll steak around vegetables and secure with tooth picks.
7. Preheat air fryer.
8. Working in batches, depending on the size of your air fryer, place bundles into basket of air fryer.
9. Spray vegetables with olive oil spray.
10. Cook at 400 degrees for 5 minutes.
11. Remove steak bundles and allow to rest for 5 minutes prior to serving/slicing.
12. WHILE steak is resting, into small-medium sauce pan heat: balsamic vinegar, stock and butter over medium heat. Whisk to combine.
13. Continue cooking until sauce has thickened and reduced by half. Season with salt and pepper.
14. Pour sauce over steak bundles prior to serving.

Nutrition
Calories: 247| Carbs: 5.6g|Protein: 30.9g|Fat: 10.9g| Sodium: 902mg | Fiber: 1.6g| Sugar:2.9g

28. Spinach Stuffed Chicken Breasts

Prep Time: 10 minutes | Cook Time: 25 minutes | Serves 4

4 chicken breasts
15ml olive oil or avocado oil
6g paprika
6g salt
1g garlic powder
2g onion powder
113g softened cream cheese
2g grated Parmesan
28g mayonnaise
45g chopped fresh spinach
2g garlic
1g red pepper flakes

Instructions
1. Preheat oven to 375 degrees.

2. Place the chicken breasts on a cutting board and drizzle with oil.

3. Add the paprika, 1/2 teaspoon salt, garlic powder, and onion powder to a small bowl and stir to combine. Sprinkle evenly over both sides of the chicken.

4. Use a sharp knife to cut a pocket into the side of each chicken breast. Set chicken aside.

5. Add cream cheese, Parmesan, mayonnaise, spinach, garlic, red pepper and remaining ½ teaspoon of salt to a small mixing bowl and stir well to combine.

6. Spoon the spinach mixture into each chicken breast evenly.

7. Place the chicken breasts in a 9x13 baking dish. Bake, uncovered, for 25-30 minutes or until chicken is cooked through.

Nutrition

Calories: 407 |Carbs: 3g |Protein: 41g| Fat: 24 | Sodium: 873mg |Fiber: 1g |Sugar: 1g

29. Pizza Flavored Keto Stuffed Tomato

Prep Time: 10 minutes | Cook Time: 8 minutes | Serves 4

- 4 slicing tomatoes
- 57g diced pepperoni finely
- 57g diced red onion finely
- 6g basil
- 6g oregano
- 6g stevia powder
- 1g coarsely ground black pepper
- 3g salt
- 64g shredded mozzarella cheese

Instruction

1. Preheat broiler on high setting.

2. Wash tomatoes and slice off the top (with the stem). Scoop out the seeds/middle of the tomato with a spoon or cut away with a paring knife. 3. Stir together spices in a small mixing bowl.

4. Stuff the middle of each tomato with a layer of onion, pepperoni, spice mixture, and cheese. Gently press down the filling with your finger and repeat the layers. You want the tomato to be slightly overfilled, as the ingredients will shrink down when the cheese melts.

5. Spray a muffin tin or square baking dish with non-stick spray. Place the tomatoes in your prepped pan.

6. Bake under the broiler for 5-8 minutes, or until the cheese and tomatoes start to brown.

Nutrition
Calories: 215 | Carbs: 5g |Protein: 13g |Fat: 16g |Sodium: 807mg |Fiber:1g | Sugar: 3g

30. Low Carb Goulash
Prep Time: 20 minutes | Cook Time: 50 minutes | Serves 3-4

½ large onion diced
4 garlic cloves sliced
454g minced beef
1 chopped carrot
3 chopped tomatoes
½ chopped green bell pepper
15ml olive oil
14g butter
27g paprika
6g cumin
6g chipotle
Salt and pepper to taste

Instructions
1. Place a heavy-bottomed pan or Dutch oven over medium heat.
2. Season the beef with salt and pepper and add to the hot pan with a tablespoon of oil.
3. Cook until fully browned, stirring to break up any clumps as needed.
4. Remove the browned meat from pan and set aside.
5. Add olive oil and butter to the pan.
6. Once the butter is melted, add the onions. Cook the onions until golden brown, or about 6-8 minutes.
7. Add the garlic, paprika, and return the beef to the pan and cook for 2 minutes.
8. Add the carrots and just enough water to cover the mixture.
9. Bring to a boil. Once boiling, reduce to a simmer, cover and cook for 45 minutes.
10. Skim off any grease that has accumulated on top.
11. Add tomatoes and peppers and cook for 5 minutes.
12. Season again with additional salt, pepper, and paprika as needed before serving.

Nutrition
Calories: 388 |Carbs: 9g |Protein: 21g|Fat: 30g |Sodium: 120mg |Fiber: 4g |Sugar: 3g

31. Egg Roll In A Bowl

Prep Time: 5 minutes | Cook Time: 10 minutes | Serves 4

- 454g minced beef
- 6g minced garlic
- 397g shredded cabbage or coleslaw mix
- 59ml low-sodium soy sauce
- 2g ground ginger
- 1 whole egg
- 8g sriracha
- 15ml sesame oil
- 28g sliced spring onions

Instructions

1. In a large skillet, brown the beef until no longer pink. Drain the meat if it's really wet.
2. Add the garlic and sautee for 30 seconds. Add the cabbage/coleslaw, soy sauce, ginger, and sautee until desired tenderness. You can add a little water if you need more liquid to sautee the coleslaw down.
3. Make a well in the center of the skillet and add the egg. Scramble until done over low heat.
4. Stir in sriracha. Drizzle with sesame oil and sprinkle with spring onions. Add additional soy sauce and sriracha if desired.

Nutrition
Calories: 331 |Carbs: 4.9g|Protein: 24.3g |Fat:23.4g |Sodium:866 mg | Fiber:1.9g

32. Red Pepper Egg-In-A-Hole

Prep Time: 5 minutes | Cook Time: 15 minutes | Serves 4

- olive oil spray
- 1 bell pepper cut into
- 4 1/2" thick rings
- 4 large eggs
- salt and fresh pepper

Instructions

1. In a large nonstick skillet, heat on medium heat.
2. When hot, spray olive oil spray, add pepper and let it cook a minute, then add egg into the center of the pepper.
3. Season with salt and pepper and cook until the egg whites are mostly set but the yolks are still runny, 2-3 minutes.

4. Gently flip and cook 1 more minute for over easy, longer if you like them over well.

Nutrition
Calories: 80 | Carbs: 1.5g | Protein: 6.5g |Fat: 5g |sodium:82 mg |Fiber: 0.5g |Sugar: 1.2g

CHAPTER 4   SNACKS

1. Keto Skillet Cookie

Prep Time: 10minutes | Cook Time: 25 minutes | Serves 8

- 200g ground almonds
- 2g baking soda
- 3g salt
- 113g butter, softened
- 64g erythritol or similar sweetener
- 1 egg
- 2ml vanilla extract
- 44g sugar-free chocolate chips

Instructions
1. Preheat the oven to 325°F and lightly grease a 10" oven-proof skillet.
2. In a medium mixing bowl, whisk together the ground almonds, salt, and baking soda.
3. In a large mixing bowl, beat butter until creamy. Add in sweetener, egg, and vanilla extract. Slowly add in bowl of dry ingredients, mixing as your pour, until well combined.
4. Stir chocolate chips into batter with a spatula or wooden spoon.
5. Scoop dough into skillet and spread to cover. Bake for 25 minutes or until the cookie is a light golden brown. The cookie will be very soft when removed from the oven.
6. Allow cookie to cool about 10-15 minutes before serving. It will continue to firm up as it cools, so wait until it cools completely to cut if serving in slices.

Nutrition
Calories: 287 | Carbs: 9g | Protein: 7g | Fat: 28g |Sodium: 323mg| Fiber: 4g | Sugar: 1g

2. Keto Strawberry Upside-Down Cake

Prep Time: 5 minutes | Cook Time: 2 minutes | Serves 2

- 14g butter

1 Egg beaten
14g sour cream
12g ground almonds
8g coconut flour
28g erythritol
5g baking powder
2g baking soda
5ml vanilla extract
43g chopped strawberries

Instructions

1. Grease two microwave safe ramekins and set aside.
2. In a mixing bowl, combine butter, egg, sour cream, ground almonds, coconut flour, granulated erythritol, baking powder, baking soda and vanilla extract. Whisk until the ingredients are completely combined.
3. Cover the bottom of each mug with a layer of chopped strawberries.
4. Divide the batter between the two mugs or ramekins, spreading evenly on top of the strawberries.
5. Microwave the mugs on high for 90 seconds. If still wet on top, microwave for an additional 20 seconds.
6. Let the mugs sit for a minute or two, then flip over onto a plate. You can also enjoy straight from the mug!

Nutrition

Calories: 163| Carbs: 7g | Protein: 5g | Fat: 13g | Sodium: 369mg |Fiber: 2g | Sugar: 2g

3. Keto Cucumber Avocado and Pomegranate Salad

Prep Time: 5 minutes | Cook Time: 5 minutes | Serves 1

1-2 chopped avocadoes
1 chopped cucumber
15ml lime juice
30ml olive oil
Salt and Pepper to taste
64g pomegranate seeds
optional garnish:coriander

Instructions

1. Combine avocados, cucumber, lime juice, and olive oil in a large mixing bowl. Toss well to coat and soften the avocados slightly.
2. Lightly season with salt and pepper. Top with pomegranate seeds and/or coriander, if Desired.

Nutrition
Calories: 112 | Carbs: 6g | Protein: 1g | Fat: 9g | Sodium: 3mg | Fiber: 3g | Sugar: 2g

4. Low Carb Blueberry Cobbler

Prep Time: 5 minutes | Cook Time: 25 minutes | Serves 2

   120g blueberries fresh or frozen
   3ml lemon juice
   1g xanthan gum
   40g ground almonds
   30g coconut flour
   30glow carb sugar substitute add more if needed
   5 eggs beaten
   19g butter melted

Instructions

1. Pour berries into a greased 9x9-inch pan.
2. Sprinkle it with lemon juice and xanthan gum. If desired, add in an additional 2-4 tablespoons of sweetener to the blueberry mixture.
3. Stir ground almonds, coconut flour, 64g granular sweetener and egg until mixture resembles coarse meal.
4. Sprinkle dry mixture over berries.
5. Drizzle melted butter over topping.
6. Bake at 350 degrees for 25 minutes or until the top is browned.

Nutrition
Calories: 103 | Carbs: 7.1g | Protein: 1.1g | Fat: 8.3g | Sodium: 62mg | Fiber: 1.2g | Sugar: 5g

5. 3-ingredient No Bake Keto Peanut Butter Balls

Prep Time: 2 minutes | Cook Time: 1 minute | Serving 20 Balls

   270g smooth peanut butter
   64g sticky sweetener of choice
   49g coconut flour

Instructions
1. Line a large tray or plate with parchment paper and set aside.

2. In a large mixing bowl, combine all your ingredients and mix well. If the batter is too thick, add some liquid (milk or water) until a thick batter remains.
3. Using your hands, form the dough into small balls and place on the lined plate/tray. Refrigerate the peanut butter and no bake balls for 30 minutes, or until firm.

Nutrition
Calories: 57 | Carbs: 3g | Protein: 2g | Fat: 4g | Sodium: 183mg | Fiber: 0.3g |Sugar: 1g

6. Keto Jalapeno Poppers
Prep Time : 10 minutes | Cook Time: 10 minutes | Yield 8 poppers

4 jalapenos
85g softened cream cheese
100g shredded cheddar
2g garlic powder
1g onion powder
4 slices bacon

Instructions
1. Slice jalapenos in half lengthwise. Carefully scrape out the seeds and membranes with a spoon and discard. See note.
2. Add the cream cheese, cheddar, garlic powder, and onion powder to a small bowl and stir well to combine.
3. Spoon the cheese evenly between the jalapenos.
4. Cut the bacon slices in half and wrap each jalapeno with a half slice of bacon.

Nutrition
Calories: 96 | Carbs: 1g |Protein: 4g|Fat: 8g | Sodium: 177mg |Fiber: 0g | Sugar: 1g

7. Easy Strawberry Banana Smoothie Bowl

Prep Time:5 minutes | Cook Time: 5 minutes | Serves 1

1 banana frozen
216g frozen strawberries
64g unsweetened coconut milk or milk of choice

Instructions
1. Combine frozen banana, frozen strawberries, and coconut milk in a blender.

2. Puree until completely smooth - the mixture should be thick. Add a touch more liquid if necessary to get it to blend completely smooth. Transfer to a bowl and add toppings as desired. Enjoy!

Nutrition

Calories: 324 | Carbs: 49.1g | Protein: 2.8g | Fat: 15.7g | Sodium: 11mg | Fiber: 8.8g | Sugar: 29.3g

8. Keto Cauliflower Wings

Prep Time: 20 minutes | Cook Time: 10 minutes | Serves 4

Crispy Cauliflower
- 1 head cauliflower
- 3 eggs beaten
- 75g ground almonds
- 75g Parmesan cheese
- 3g garlic powder
- 1g smoked paprika
- Salt and Pepper to taste

Sauce
- 236ml Frank's Red Hot Sauce
- 56g butter

Instructions

1. Preheat your air fryer to 400 degrees or oven to 420.
2. Core the cauliflower and cut into larger florets.
3. Beat the eggs together in a small bowl.
4. In a separate bowl, combine the ground almonds, Parmesan, garlic powder, smoked paprika, salt and pepper.
5. Dip the cauliflower into the egg mixture, and then coat in the ground almonds mixture.
6. Transfer to a parchment lined baking sheet until ready to cook.
7. Continue with the remaining cauliflower.
8. Spray the bottom of your air fryer or a parchment lined baking sheet with oil.
9. Add the cauliflower in a single layer. Spray the top.
10. Cook for 10 to 12 minutes in the air fryer or 20 to 22 minutes in the oven, until golden brown, flipping halfway through.

Sauce

11. While the cauliflower is cooking, make the sauce by combining the Franks Hot Sauce and butter in a small saucepan.

12. Heat over medium low heat until the butter melts.

To Combine

13. Toss the crispy cauliflower with the sauce, and serve using a slotted spoon.

Nutrition

Calories: 257 | Carbs: 9g | Protein: 13g | Fat: 20g | Sodium: 1545mg | Fiber: 4g | Sugar: 3g

9. Keto No Bake Peanut Butter And Jelly Bars

Prep Time: 10 minutes | Refrigeration Time: 2 hrs | Servings: 2 bars

168g ground almonds
8g icing monkfruit/erythritol sweetener
pinch of cinnamon
1g salt
90g natural peanut butter
30g sugar free maple syrup
1g water if needed
60g no sugar added strawberry jam

Instructions

1. In a bowl, mix together all of your dry ingredients.
2. Add the peanut butter, sugar free maple syrup and water if needed, stir until a crumbly dough forms.
3. Line a loaf pan with parchment paper and press half of the dough into the pan. Press firmly enough to form an even layer.
4. Top this layer with the jam, spread evenly.
5. For the final layer, gently press chunks of this dough on top of the jelly layer until the jelly is fully covered. This layer doesn't have to look perfect! Just make sure it's pressed down enough to form a layer. (You can also take chunks of the peanut butter dough and press them together in your hand to form flattened pieces, then place those pieces on top of the jelly layer, one at a time until you can form one solid layer and press all the pieces together).
6. Refrigerate the peanut butter and jelly bars for at least 2-3 hours.
7. Lift them from the pan using parchment paper then slice into bars and serve. Enjoy!

Nutrition

Calories: 212 |Carbs: 5.5g| Protein: 7.6g | Fat: 16.5g | sodium: 427mg| Fiber: 1g| Sugar:1g

CHAPTER 5 APPETIZERS

1. Easy & Creamy Hot Crab Dip

Prep Time: 15minutes | Cook Time: 30 minutes | Serves 12

- 227g package cream cheese, softened
- 4 green onions, thinly sliced
- 113g mayonnaise
- 59ml milk
- 2 cans (170g each) lump crabmeat, drained
- 0.6g teaspoon garlic powder

Instructions
1. Preheat oven to 350°F. Lightly grease a 1-quart baking dish.
2. In a medium bowl, beat cream cheese with a mixer on medium speed until smooth. Add mayonnaise, milk, and garlic powder; beat until well combined.
3. Stir in crabmeat and green onions. Pour mixture into prepared dish.
4. Bake for 30 minutes or until bubbly. Serve with crackers, chips, or vegetables.

Nutrition
Calories: 247 | Carbs: 5g | Protein: 12g | Fat: 23g |Sodium: 506mg| Fiber: 0g | Sugar: 3g

2. Low Carb Nachos

Prep Time: 10minutes | Cook Time: 15 minutes | Serves 2

- 227g package cream cheese, softened
- 113g ground beef, cooked and crumbled
- 59ml taco sauce
- 30ml salsa
- 1g-2g chili powder
- 85g cheddar cheese, shredded
- 60g sour cream

Instructions
1. Preheat oven to 350° F. Grease a small baking dish.
2. In a medium bowl, mix together cooked beef, taco sauce, salsa, and chili powder.
3. Spread mixture evenly in the baking dish. Sprinkle with cheese.
4. Bake for 15 minutes or until cheese is melted and bubbly.
5. Serve with sour cream and additional salsa, if desired.

Nutrition
Calories: 587 | Carbs: 7g | Protein: 42g | Fat: 45g |Sodium: 1042mg| Fiber: 1g | Sugar: 3g

3. Keto Buffalo Chicken Dip

Prep Time: 5 minutes | Cook Time: 15 minutes | Serves 12

   113g cream cheese, softened
   59ml Frank's RedHot sauce
   114g blue cheese dressing
   170g cooked and shredded chicken

Instructions
1. Preheat oven to 350° F. Grease a 1-quart baking dish.
2. In a medium bowl, beat cream cheese with a mixer on medium speed until smooth.
3. Add Frank's RedHot sauce and blue cheese dressing; mix until well combined.
4. Stir in chicken. Pour mixture into prepared dish.
5. Bake for 15 minutes or until bubbly. Serve with crackers, chips, or vegetables.

Nutrition
Calories: 209 | Carbs: 4g | Protein: 10g | Fat: 17g |Sodium: 1042mg| Fiber:0g| Sugar: 2g

4. Keto Jalapeño Poppers

Prep Time: 10 minutes | Cook Time: 20 minutes | Serves 12

   6 large jalapeños, halved and seeded
   113g cream cheese, softened
   30ml shredded cheddar cheese
   1 egg, beaten
   59ml almond flour

Instructions
1. Preheat oven to 350° F. Grease a baking sheet.
2. In a medium bowl, beat cream cheese with a mixer on medium speed until smooth. Stir in cheddar cheese and egg.
3. Place almond flour in a shallow dish.
4. Stuff each jalapeño half with cream cheese mixture. Dip in almond flour to coat.
5. Place on prepared baking sheet. Bake for 20 minutes or until golden brown.
6. Serve with ranch dressing or sour cream, if desired.

Nutrition
Calories: 107 | Carbs:3g | Protein: 5g | Fat: 10g |Sodium: 143mg| Fiber:1g| Sugar: 1g

5. Low Carb Deviled Eggs

Prep Time: 15 minutes | Cook Time: 10 minutes | Serves 6

- 6 eggs, hard-boiled and cooled
- 59ml mayonnaise
- 15ml yellow mustard
- 30ml pickle juice
- Salt and pepper, to taste

Instructions
1. Cut eggs in half lengthwise. Remove yolks and place in a medium bowl.
2. Add mayonnaise, yellow mustard, pickle juice, salt, and pepper to the bowl with the yolks. Mash with a fork until smooth.
3. Spoon or pipe mixture into egg whites.
4. Serve immediately or store in the refrigerator for later. Enjoy!

Nutrition
Calories: 90 | Carbs: 1g | Protein: 6g | Fat: 7g |Sodium: 147mg| Fiber: 0g| Sugar: 1g

6. Low Carb Rangoon

Prep Time: 10 minutes | Cook Time: 20 minutes | Serves 12

- 85g cream cheese, softened
- 113g crab meat
- 1 green onion, finely chopped
- 1 egg, beaten
- 35g almond flour

Instructions
1. Preheat oven to 350° F. Line a baking sheet with parchment paper.
2. In a medium bowl, mix together cream cheese, crab meat, green onion, and egg.
3. Place almond flour in a shallow dish.
4. Using your hands, form the mixture into 12 small balls. Dip in almond flour to coat.
5. Place on prepared baking sheet. Bake for 20 minutes or until golden brown.
6. Serve with sweet and sour sauce or cocktail sauce, if desired.
7. Enjoy!

Nutrition

Calories: 90 | Carbs: 1g | Protein: 5g | Fat: 7g |Sodium: 143mg| Fiber: 0g| Sugar: 1g

7. Low-carb Cheese Sticks

Prep Time: 5 minutes | Cook Time: 10 minutes | Yields 12 cheese sticks

   85g mozzarella cheese, shredded
   14g Parmesan cheese, grated
   1 egg, beaten
   113g almond flour
   4g garlic powder
   1g onion powder
   1g dried oregano
   1g dried basil
   3g salt

Instructions

1. Preheat oven to 400° F. Line a baking sheet with parchment paper.
2. In a medium bowl, mix together mozzarella cheese, Parmesan cheese, egg, and almond flour. Stir in garlic powder, onion powder, oregano, basil, and salt.
3. Roll mixture into 12 balls. Place on prepared baking sheet and press down slightly to flatten.
4. Bake for 10 minutes or until golden brown.
5. Serve with marinara sauce or your favorite dipping sauce.

Nutrition

Calories: 207 | Carbs: 7g | Protein: 10g | Fat: 16g |Sodium: 606mg| Fiber: 2g| Sugar: 1g

8. Easy Cheesy Courgette Breadsticks

Prep Time: 10 minutes | Cook Time: 20 minutes | Serves 4

   1 large courgette, shredded
   85g cheddar cheese, shredded
   113g almond flour
   1 egg, beaten
   1g salt
   1g baking powder

Instructions

1. Preheat oven to 400° F. Grease a baking sheet.
2. In a medium bowl, mix together zucchini, cheese, almond flour, egg, salt, and baking powder until well combined.
3. Drop dough by spoonfuls onto the prepared baking sheet.
4. Bake for 20 minutes or until golden brown.
5. Serve with marinara sauce or your favorite dipping sauce.

Nutrition

Calories: 572 | Carbs: 20g | Protein: 36g | Fat: 45g |Sodium: 1343mg| Fiber: 5g| Sugar: 7g

Appendix 1 Measurement Conversion Chart

MEASUREMENT CONVERSION CHART

VOLUME EQUIVALENTS (DRY)

US STANDARD	METRIC (APPROXIMATE)
1/8 teaspoon	0.5 mL
1/4 teaspoon	1 mL
1/2 teaspoon	2 mL
3/4 teaspoon	4 mL
1 teaspoon	5 mL
1 tablespoon	15 mL
1/4 cup	59 mL
1/2 cup	118 mL
3/4 cup	177 mL
1 cup	235 mL
2 cups	475 mL
3 cups	700 mL
4 cups	1 L

VOLUME EQUIVALENTS (LIQUID)

US STANDARD	US STANDARD (OUNCES)	METRIC (APPROXIMATE)
2 tablespoons	1 fl.oz.	30 mL
1/4 cup	2 fl.oz.	60 mL
1/2 cup	4 fl.oz.	120 mL
1 cup	8 fl.oz.	240 mL
1 1/2 cup	12 fl.oz.	355 mL
2 cups or 1 pint	16 fl.oz.	475 mL
4 cups or 1 quart	32 fl.oz.	1 L
1 gallon	128 fl.oz.	4 L

TEMPERATURES EQUIVALENTS

FAHRENHEIT(F)	CELSIUS(C) (APPROXIMATE)
225 °F	107 °C
250 °F	120 °C
275 °F	135 °C
300 °F	150 °C
325 °F	160 °C
350 °F	180 °C
375 °F	190 °C
400 °F	205 °C
425 °F	220 °C
450 °F	235 °C
475 °F	245 °C
500 °F	260 °C

WEIGHT EQUIVALENTS

US STANDARD	METRIC (APPROXIMATE)
1 ounce	28 g
2 ounces	57 g
5 ounces	142 g
10 ounces	284 g
15 ounces	425 g
16 ounces (1 pound)	455 g
1.5 pounds	680 g
2 pounds	907 g

Appendix 2 Measurement Conversion Chart

The Dirty Dozen and Clean Fifteen

The Environmental Working Group (EWG) is a nonprofit, nonpartisan organization dedicated to protecting human health and the environment Its mission is to empower people to live healthier lives in a healthier environment. This organization publishes an annual list of the twelve kinds of produce, in sequence, that have the highest amount of pesticide residue-the Dirty Dozen-as well as a list of the fifteen kinds of produce that have the least amount of pesticide residue-the Clean Fifteen.

THE DIRTY DOZEN

- The 2016 Dirty Dozen includes the following produce. These are considered among the year's most important produce to buy organic:

Strawberries	Spinach
Apples	Tomatoes
Nectarines	Bell peppers
Peaches	Cherry tomatoes
Celery	Cucumbers
Grapes	Kale/collard greens
Cherries	Hot peppers

- The Dirty Dozen list contains two additional items kale/collard greens and hot peppers-because they tend to contain trace levels of highly hazardous pesticides.

THE CLEAN FIFTEEN

- The least critical to buy organically are the Clean Fifteen list. The following are on the 2016 list:

Avocados	Papayas
Corn	Kiw
Pineapples	Eggplant
Cabbage	Honeydew
Sweet peas	Grapefruit
Onions	Cantaloupe
Asparagus	Cauliflower
Mangos	

- Some of the sweet corn sold in the United States are made from genetically engineered (GE) seedstock. Buy organic varieties of these crops to avoid GE produce.

Printed in Great Britain
by Amazon